AQUA AEROBICS
A Scientific Approach

D1279378

by

Tom Kinder
Professor of Physical Education
and Athletic Director
Bridgewater College
Bridgewater, VA

Julie See
National Aqua Aerobics Instructor

Jennifer Phillips Webster
Illustrator

eddie bowers publishing, inc.
2600 Jackson Street
Dubuque, IA 52001

eddie bowers publishing, inc.
2600 Jackson Street
Dubuque, Iowa 52001

ISBN 0-945483-20-1

Printed in the United States of America.

9 8 7 6 5 4 3 2 1

TABLE OF CONTENTS

CHAPTER 2
SAFETY 17

CHAPTER 3
CONDUCTING CLASS 37

CHAPTER 4
THE OLDER/MATURE ADULT 79

CHAPTER 5
EQUIPMENT 91

PREFACE

This book is written to introduce the physical educator, the wellness advocator, the aquatics personnel, the mature adult, and the student to a different approach to water exercises. Throughout this book there is a consciousness of the necessities of safety. At one time or another all of us have dealt with a situation that has forced us to focus personally on some issue of concern. Water and water activities can be safe and fun when a person minimizes the risks from hazards that he or she may face. This book was prepared with this in mind.

It is firmly believed that happiness, well being, and the will-to-live result from active participation, not from passive observation. Values accrue to an activity when the individual can gain status through the thrill of accomplishment, no matter the size of the advancement or the age of the participant.

The information in this book is based upon science. There is new data that has been incorporated into aqua aerobics for the 90's. This book contains cross training activities, elderhostel activities and aerobics fitness activities. There are also formats for conducting classes - some using music.

There was a need to have an appropriate written source in the area of aqua aerobics. There is little written information available for preparing educators in this growing specialty.

ACKNOWLEDGEMENTS

My thanks are gratefully extended to the publisher, Eddie Bowers, and his staff who make publishing quality material a priority for their profession.

A special recognition is extended to the outstanding professional art work of Jennifer Phillips Webster and recognition to her husband Jon for sharing her with us. Jennifer conceptualized and prepared all illustrations for this book.

The assistance of Julie See, who carried out much of the research and preliminary work on this text should be acknowledged. Julie was involved in a great deal of travel in order to bring ideas together for this project. Thanks are extended to her husband Craig for his constant support and encouragement.

Julie See wishes to acknowledge and thank Ruth Sova and the Aquatic Exercise Association for providing the theoretical information and practical experience upon which this book is based.

I also would like to extend my appreciation to Ellen K. Layman, the Director of Public Information at Bridgewater College and a true professional, for carefully and skillfully synthesizing our individual writing styles, making valuable suggestions, and critically reviewing parts of the manuscript.

Finally, I owe a particular debt of gratitude to my wife Debra and our two daughters, Mandy and Marsha, who gave me the idea for putting together this text. We all acknowledge the support we have received from a much higher source than is humanly possible.

T.M.K.

ABOUT THE CONTRIBUTORS

Julie See

Julie has certifications from
IDEA   -- Certified professonial aerobics instructor, Gold Certificate
AFAA   -- Certified professonial aerobics instructor
AEA   -- Certified professional aquatics exercise instructor
AEA   -- Aquatics Training Specialist

She has been in demand for professional training workshops throughout the country and in Japan. The following are some examples for just 1990-92.

America's Fitness Conference, Milwaukee, WI
Mini Mania Convention, Chicago, IL
Midwest Mania, Chicago, IL
Dallas Mania, Dallas, TX
International Aquatic Fitness Conference (IAFC), Chicago, IL
1st Water Exercise Conference, Japan
IAFC, San Diego, CA
AEA Regional Conferences, various locations
Fitness Network, The Palms Resorts, Palm Springs, CA

Julie was presented the 1991 Outstanding Fitness Instructor Award at the International Aquatic and Fitness Conference in San Diego, California. She has written many articles, the most recent being "Aqua Power Aerobics." She runs her own Fitness Center in Petersburg, West Virginia.

Jennifer Phillips Webster

Jennifer is a professional artist presently located in Columbia, South Carolina. She has illustrated numerous books. She worked on *Organizational Management Administration for Athletic Programs* by *eddie bowers publishing, inc.* in both 1987 and 1990. She has painted many outstanding water color pictures which have been sold in galleries throughout Virginia.

Dr. Thomas M. Kinder

Tom is a Professor and Chair of the Physical Education Department and Athletic Director at Bridgewater College, Bridgewater, Virginia. He is the author and editor of *Organizational Management Administration for Athletic Programs* now in its second edition. He has written numerous articles and has served on the editorial board of several publications.

His most recent publication was an article for the Salem Press on Sam Huff. This was done for a children sports encyclopedia.

He also has been involved in many national organizations. He has served as a member of the N.C.A.A. Council and on various N.C.A.A. committees.

Chapter 1

GENERAL INFORMATION

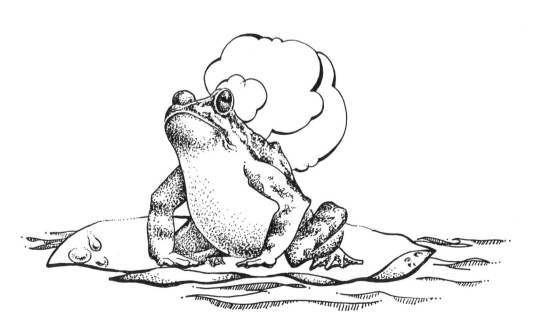

EXERCISE PRINCIPLES

COMPONENTS

Physical fitness has five major components: flexibility, muscular strength, muscular endurance, cardio-respiratory endurance, and body composition. Therefore, a well-rounded fitness program should provide a means of improving each of these components; aquatic aerobic exercise when properly performed meets this goal.

Flexibility

Flexibility is the range of motion that a limb can move; movement always occurs at a joint. With the lessened effect of gravity and the comfortable environment, water allows most people to move through their full range of motion with more ease. Flexibility can be increased by proper techniques which include both static stretches and rhythmic limbering movements. A static stretch is a sustained stretch and provides safer, more effective results than ballistic stretches (bouncing) which can cause microscopic tears within the muscle.

Muscular Strength

Muscular strength is the ability of a muscle to exert a maximal force in a single repetition. Strength gains are seen when the demands upon the muscles are systematically increased through greater resistance. Because water has a greater density than air it provides for at least 12 times the resistance, thus increasing demands upon the muscular system. This increased demand leads to strength gains, especially notable in the beginning participant. Once a person's muscular system has adapted to water exercise, strength gains will plateau; in order to see further gains, resistance equipment can be incorporated into the program.

Muscular Endurance

Muscular endurance is the ability of a muscle to exert submaximal force for several repetitions. Improvements in muscular endurance are seen when performing an exercise for more than 15 repetitions. Therefore, aquatic aerobic exercise lends itself well to increasing endurance as the basic movements are repeated many times throughout the exercise period.

Cardio-Respiratory Endurance

Cardio-respiratory endurance is the ability of the heart and lungs to supply oxygenated blood throughout the muscles of the body. Aerobic exercise provides training for the cardio-respiratory system by strengthening the heart and lungs and increasing their capacity to do the required work. The movements typically found in the aerobic portion of an aquatic exercise program, such as jogging, leaping and jumping, all provide effective means of overloading the cardio-respiratory system.

Body Composition

Body composition is the ratio of body fat to lean body mass. This is not a matter of being overweight, rather being "overfat," as muscle tissue is more dense, and thus weighs more, than fat. To improve the body composition, it is most effective to perform a low intensity, long duration aerobic program in conjunction with modifying dietary intake. Aquatic aerobic exercise is ideal in that the heart rates are lower and the impact is lessened as compared to the same program performed on land. This allows for one to continue for a longer period of time and thus a greater percentage of fat calories will be consumed.

TRAINING PRINCIPLES

In order to develop and maintain a well-rounded fitness program, several principles should be remembered and applied.

Progressive Overload

To gain improvements in any system of the body, the demands to that system must be increased or overloaded. So that training (adaptation) occurs rather than injury, it is imperative that the demands be applied in increments that the body can handle. This is known as progressive overload.

Specificity

Specificity refers to the need to train a system, or a muscle group, in a certain manner to achieve the desired results. Strength training requires increased resistance and differs from endurance training which requires increased repetitions. Abdominal exercises will not provide strength gains in the triceps muscle. A toning class will not develop cardio-respiratory endurance. A distance runner does not train for competition by running only fast sprints. One must design a specific fitness program to meet the desired goals.

Variability

However, if we always train in exactly the same manner, for the same length of time, the same number of days on the same days of the week, we ignore the principle of variability. Not only will we become weary of our program, but stressing the body repeatedly in the same way can lead to overuse injuries. It is enjoyable, and effective, to vary the type of program (cross-training), the length and intensity of individual workouts, the frequency of training each week, and the specific exercises performed.

Reversibility

Fitness cannot be stored. One cannot train for six weeks and expect to retain the goals achieved without continuing a maintenance program; it is often said that it takes 12 weeks to get into shape but only two weeks to get out of shape. This is the principle of reversibility. The body adapts to progressive overload with improvements to the system in training, but if this overload is removed, the body will revert back to the previous condition. In other words, "if you don't use it, you'll lose it" applies to fitness; it needs to become a lifelong habit.

THE ACSM GUIDELINES

The American College of Sports Medicine (ACSM) has updated its position statement for developing/maintaining cardio-respiratory fitness and proper body composition in healthy adults. This statement makes recommendations on frequency, intensity, duration and mode of aerobic activity as well as the inclusion of resistance training. The activity must utilize the large muscle groups of the body, be rhythmical and performed continuously for 20 to 60 minutes at the proper intensity (50-85% maximum oxygen uptake) three to five times per week. Moderate intensity strength training is also recommended for a minimum of two days per week with eight to 10 exercises for the major muscle groups of the body (eight to 12 repetitions per exercise).

Intensity of aerobic activity can be most effectively monitored by maximum oxygen uptake (VO max); however this necessitates the use of a spirometer which measures the breathing capacity of the lungs.

However, few exercise facilities have access to this equipment so other methods are utilized in a class setting to give a close approximation. These methods will be more fully discussed in Chapter 3.

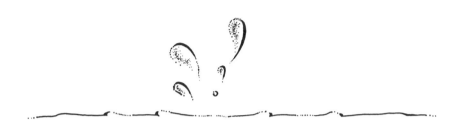

PHYSICAL LAWS OF WATER

BUOYANCY

The physical qualities of water create a much different exercise medium than air. As discussed previously, water has a greater density than air and therefore provides more resistance to movement. The human body is also buoyant in water; the degree of buoyancy depends upon the actual body composition and the amount of air held in the lungs. The force of buoyancy (which applies an upward pressure on a submerged body) is somewhat less than the force of gravity. Buoyancy causes the impact of the foot coming in contact with the ground while the body is partially submerged in water to be greatly reduced as compared to a similar exercise performed on land. The deeper the water, the less the impact because submerged objects effectively weigh less than on land; it is generally stated that when submerged to neck depth, you weigh only 10% of your land weight.

Sir Isaac Newton, the English mathematician and natural philosopher, worked extensively with the forces of gravity and the laws of motion. Newton's Laws of Motion have application in every phenomenon we observe including aquatic exercise, and a basic understanding of these laws will help to develop a more effective program. The three principles which govern the motion of all material objects are listed below.

INERTIA

Law 1. An object remains at rest or in a state of uniform motion unless acted on by a force.

ACCELERATION

Law 2. The reaction of the body as measured by its acceleration is proportional to the force applied and inversely proportional to the mass.

ACTION/REACTION

Law 3. For every action there is an equal and opposite reaction.

CHANGING INTENSITY LEVEL

It is obviously very important to be knowledgeable in various ways of modifying the intensity of any given exercise or workout. This will enable the program to be designed to fit individual needs, thus making the program more effective.

LAWS OF MOTION

Inertia (Law 1) is exemplified in exercise by the fact that it is easier - takes less force - to remain at rest than it does to begin moving. It also takes less force to continue moving in the same direction than to change direction, or to continue the same movement rather than change to another exercise. For example, it is easier to stand in the water than it is to begin jogging; it is easier to jog forward for eight counts than to jog forward four counts and then back four counts; and it is easier to continue jogging than to jog eight counts, kick front eight counts, then jump eight counts. Therefore to increase the intensity of a workout by utilizing the principle of inertia, simply incorporate more change (stopping and starting, changing direction or mode of movement) which will require more force to be exerted.

Acceleration (Law 2) allows for another method of intensity change. An individual's mass (body weight/gravity) will not alter during the workout, but the force applied can vary throughout. By encouraging participants to jump higher, leap further, and pull harder, they will increase the force applied to move their body mass through the water, and the intensity of the workout will proportionally increase. It is also important to consider the principle of acceleration when comparing participants. As an example, if one student weighs 100 pounds and another weighs 150 pounds, but both exert the same amount of force while leaping through the water, the 100-pound student will propel through the water faster. Encourage participants to perform as individuals; each has unique goals and abilities.

The principle of action/reaction (Law 3) is easily visualized in aquatic exercise: when you push your feet down onto the pool bottom, your body will move upwards toward the surface, and when you scoop the hands and pull the water toward the left, you facilitate movement of the body toward the right. By incorporating this principle, arm movements can either assist or impede the movement of the body. When jogging forward, if you use a forward crawl motion of the arms, you will assist the movement of the body through the water. But if you use a back crawl motion with the arms, you will impede the forward motion of the body through the water. This knowledge allows for movements to be more efficient in reaching specific goals.

PRINCIPLE OF LEVER ARM

Muscular contraction causes movement at the joints (the articulation of two or more bones). The human body can be visualized as a system of levers; levers are defined as a bar (bone) turning about a fixed point (joint). A lever has three points which determine which type of lever it is and for what motion it is best suited. The point of rotation, or fulcrum, is the joint of the body where the movement occurs; the point of force application is usually the insertion of the muscle which contracts to produce the movement; the point of resistance application is sometimes the center of gravity of the lever and sometimes the location of an external resistance. When working in the water, the resistance becomes the amount of water displaced by the lever when movement is produced; in effect, water is an external resistance just as a dumbbell would be when exercising on land.

Most of the levers of the human body are third class levers where the force is located on the same side of the fulcrum as the resistance. Typically a third class lever is designed for speed and range of motion; therefore, a great deal of force is required to move even a small resistance. A true example of third class leverage is the brachialis contracting concentrically to flex the forearm (bend the elbow). The elbow is the fulcrum; the brachialis inserts on the ulna just below the

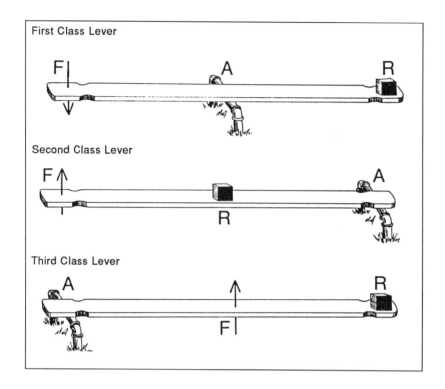

First Class Lever

Second Class Lever

Third Class Lever

elbow and is the point of force application, and the water displaced by the movement of the forearm is the resistance. Since the ulna cannot rotate, the pull is direct and true.

The following formula explains the relationship of the length of the lever arms. Force arm is the distance between the joint and the muscle insertion and resistance arm is the distance between the joint and the point of resistance application.

Force X Force Arm = Resistance X Resistance Arm

When exercising in the water, we can use the principles of levers to change the intensity of an exercise - the longer the resistance arm, the more difficult the exercise becomes. For example, a kneelift is easier to perform than a straight leg lift to the front, although the action at the joint is the same (concentric contraction of the iliopsoas to lift the leg). Because the force arm will remain constant while the resistance arm and the amount of water displaced changes, the force exerted will vary. This allows for individual modification of intensity without changing the exercise performed.

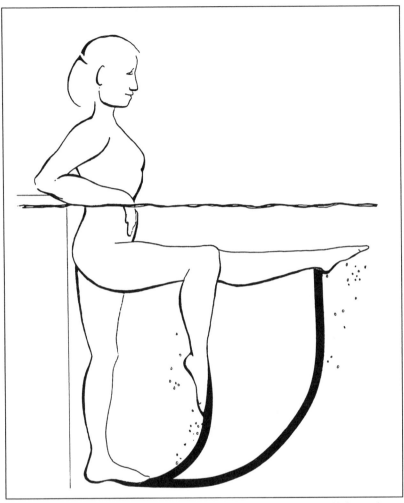

Changing intensity by altering length of resistance arm; a kneelift is easier to perform than a straight leg lift to the front.

EDDY DRAG

Whenever an object moves through the water (or water moves around an object), currents are created; in very simplified terms, this is eddy drag. Eddy drag is a principle well-recognized by swimmers, who wish to create a streamlined body to minimize the amount of drag because it hinders speed of movement. However, in aquatic exercise one may want to employ eddy drag to increase the benefits of the workout.

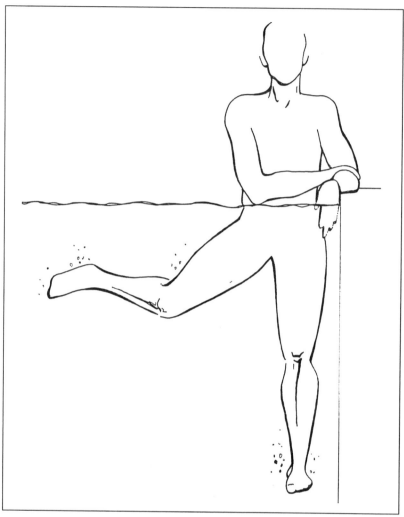

An example of utilizing Eddy Drag to increase resistance; slightly flexing the knee during a side leg lift.

When performing a side leg lift, if the participant keeps the leg fully extended (not hyperextended which is unsafe) at the knee, the water will offer a certain amount of resistance. If the same exercise is performed with the knee slightly flexed, more eddy drag is created and the exercise intensity is increased. Note: this a different principle than length of resistance arm; the knee in this case is only slightly flexed and therefore the length is not changed significantly. For a range of intensity levels when performing a side leg lift, one would bend the knee fully (short resistance arm) for the easiest workout, straighten the leg for a intermediate workout, and slightly flex the knee to increase eddy drag (but maintain a long resistance arm) for the most difficult workout. This will utilize two different principles for intensity change.

FRONTAL SURFACE

The more surface area moved through the water, the more water must be displaced and the more intense the activity becomes. It will be easier to walk sideways through the water than to walk forward, because the surface area of the body moving forward is greater. This can be seen by comparing the silhouette of the body from a front view and a side view. The frontal surface can be further increased when walking forward by rotating the arms outward so the palms face forward. A simple, but very effective, method of changing intensity of the workout is hand positioning. By keeping the hand flat and slicing through the water, frontal surface area is minimal and the intensity is low. Making a fist will increase the frontal surface and the intensity, and by pulling the water with a slightly cupped hand the workload becomes even

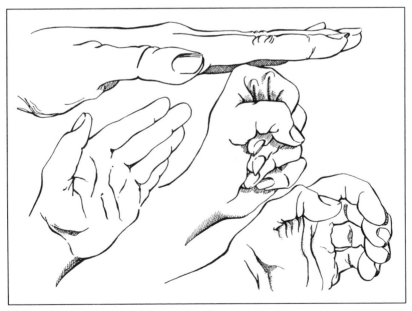

Various hand positions which can alter the intensity of an exercise.

greater. Again, this allows participants to perform the same movement, or exercise, with individual modifications in intensity.

USE OF EQUIPMENT

Water exercise equipment is extremely varied, not only in cost, but in purpose and design. Because equipment will be more fully discussed in a later chapter, it will suffice to say that by magnifying the principles discussed above, the use of equipment can increase the intensity of an aquatic workout.

SPEED OF EXECUTION

We are now aware that the density of water provides more resistance, so it is only natural that this creates a decreased speed of execution of movements.

LAND SPEED vs WATER SPEED

Try to visualize how it feels to jog through a pool filled with water; then imagine the pool filled with molasses and finally filled with tar. All three media are liquid, but the density of each is different and the speed of movement will be proportionally impacted. A similar situation occurs when comparing movements on land to the same movements in the water; water necessitates slower execution of movement. This is not a problem in itself, but if an instructor does not take into consideration the difference between land speed and water speed, complications will arise.

Execution of aquatic exercise can be divided into fast speed and slow speed; fast speed allows for the heart rate to be elevated into the target zone, while slow speeds allow for full range of motion (ROM) of the joints. By incorporating both into a single workout, a better balance is maintained and one can work aerobically without compromising flexibility. Even fast water speed is slower than land speed. If it were to take a single count to perform a kneelift on land, it would take two counts to perform at fast water speed, and four counts at slow water speed. Both feet will come in contact with the pool bottom between repetitions when working at slow water speed - either with a bounce, or by stepping in place or bending at the knees if lowered impact is required.

CUEING

A period of time elapses from when the brain receives a signal to when the body actually is able to perform that command - your reaction time. As an example, when you see the brake lights of the car in front of you, a matter of seconds will elapse before you can transfer your foot from the gas pedal to the brake pedal and stop your car. A similar response is seen when participating in an exercise class; the instructor will give a command, verbal and/or non-verbal, to change, and it will take a period of time to successfully negotiate the command. The actual reaction will depend upon the degree of change required as well as the individual's abilities. Because speed of movement is decelerated in the water, reaction time to the same command will be slower than on land. To make transitions more effective and safe, it becomes necessary to give cues earlier when teaching aquatic exercise. There is no right or wrong way to cue for transitions, but effectiveness is easily monitored through observation of class participants. Beginners and less physically fit individuals will usually require more reaction time to make transitions.

It is likely that more injuries occur during transitions than in specific movements or exercises, as the body is often temporarily in a compromised position. So, reaction time is a very important concept to understand, and proper cueing is a very important technique to master. A class that is easy to follow is also much more enjoyable for participants.

WATER DEPTH

As water depth increases, impact decreases because the effect of gravitational pull on the body is reduced as more of the body becomes submerged. If minimum impact to the body during exercise is a primary goal, the participant should work at the deepest possible level where control of movement can still be maintained. General recommendations for shallow water aerobic exercise is a water depth which is waist to arm-pit deep. While exercising in this range, one will be buoyant enough to lessen the impact on the joints, but will maintain enough body weight so as not to lose contact with the pool bottom and feel as if he or she were floating away. This depth also will enable the exerciser to receive toning benefits to upper body muscles because the arms can be moved through the resistive medium of the water throughout the class. Also, when working at waist to armpit depth, one can more effectively modify the intensity of the workout by incorporating a variety of arm movements.

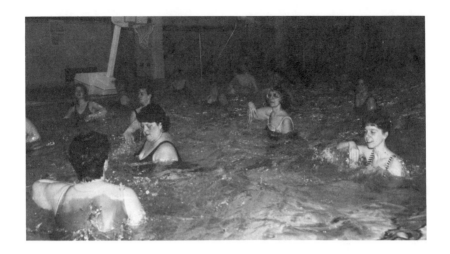

Another water exercise alternative is a deep water program; here the feet never strike the pool bottom and the workout is considered non-impact. Deep water programs are quite diverse and can be very demanding physically; however the workouts also can be designed for beginner level. In almost all cases, it will be necessary to utilize some form of equipment for a deep water exercise program to provide the buoyancy and stability to remain in an upright position. This can be accomplished through use of buoyant belts, vests, ankle cuffs or hand-held equipment. Some deep water programs do not use equipment and require that participants tread water throughout the class to remain upright; this would not be advisable, or comfortable, for non-swimmers or less conditioned individuals. Deep water programs allow for efficient use of pool time as programs can be conducted in both the shallow area and the diving area simultaneously. Although most are held in the diving well, one could technically perform a deep water program at a depth slightly less than one's height because the head will always remain out of the water. (If a participant is 5'6", he or she could execute a deep water class in about 5' of water with the use of buoyant equipment.)

WATER TEMPERATURE

Water temperature is of concern, not only for comfort but for safety. Water exercisers typically prefer the water to be slightly warmer than lap swimmers; a range of 80-84 degrees Fahrenheit is generally suggested. Even at this temperature, the water will feel cold upon entering and thus requires the participants to begin a workout with a thorough warmup to elevate the body temperature.

If the water temperature is in the lower 70s and the class is to be held, it will be necessary to spend more time in the thermal warmup phase of class to prepare the joints and muscles and prevent them from being injured. At this temperature, the muscles will tend to contract, and it is not advisable to exercise or stretch a "cold" muscle. The aerobic phase probably should be lengthened and kept as vigorous as possible, whereas the toning, and definitely the final stretch, should be significantly shortened or conducted on the deck. If it is necessary to exercise in water of this temperature, additional clothing will help to keep the body warm. A non-aerobic class, such as a toning or stretch class, should not be held in water that is this cold because the body will not remain warm enough to prevent injuries.

On the other hand, if water temperature is in the 90s, other dangers arise. The body will not be able to effectively dissipate heat created during vigorous exercise, and heat-related injuries can develop. These problems are compounded by the surrounding air temperature and humidity, and, if exercising outside, the sun's rays and the amount of air flow. Although heat cramps, heat exhaustion, and heat stroke are situations more likely to impact an instructor teaching from the deck, if the water temperature is extremely high, the participants could suffer as well. Water normally cools the body more effectively than air, but when water temperature approaches body temperature, the cooling capacity is greatly reduced. If classes are to be held in water that is excessively warm, it would be advisable to avoid aerobic type activities which only elevate body temperature. Gentle water walking, toning, and stretching classes might be suitable, but caution participants about becoming overheated and make sure to increase water consumption before, during, and after exercising.

REFERENCES

Trefil, James. *A Scientist at the Seashore*. New York: Charles Scribner's Sons, 1984.

Thompson, Clem W. *Manual of Structural Kinesiology, 11th Edition*. St. Louis: Times Mirror/Mosby Publishing, 1989.

The Aquatic Exercise Association Instructor Certification Program, Aquatic Exercise Association, Port Washington, WI.

Chapter 2

SAFETY

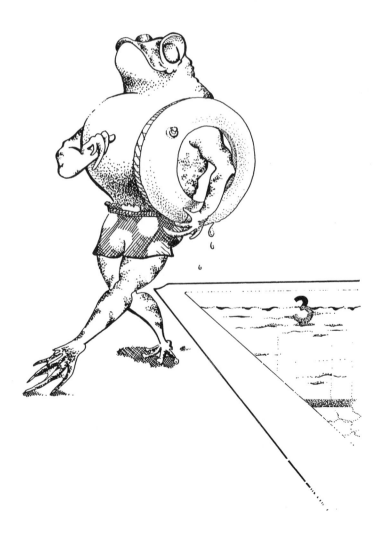

BASIC WATER SAFETY

Safety should always be the first priority in any exercise class; the instructor is responsible for the safety of every participant. Our legal system assumes that an instructor is sufficiently trained and knowledgeable about possible hazards which could arise from an exercise program. As in all situations, the best alternative is to eliminate hazards and prevent accidents; however, should an accident occur, the instructor must be able to deal with the situation calmly and efficiently. Proper training and certification are very important to prepare the instructor.

This chapter is not attempting to provide an instructor with the necessary knowledge on safety techniques. Rather, it is a quick overview of some of the most basic ideas the instructor should have before teaching the first class. The authors believe that an aquatic exercise instructor should have at least the following credentials: water exercise instructor certification, CPR certification, standard first aid training, and basic water safety training.

NEED FOR CPR TRAINING

It is necessary that all exercise instructors be certified and competent in performing Cardio-Pulmonary Resuscitation (CPR). CPR is a method of circulating oxygenated blood throughout the body of a person whose heart is not functioning; for example, someone who has suffered a heart attack. This life-saving technique is not difficult to learn, but it should be reviewed and updated periodically. (If you need further information on learning CPR, contact your local American Red Cross or American Heart Association chapter.) As an instructor, you may want to provide the opportunity for your class participants to become CPR certified. Many lives can be saved if more people have this training. Please note: CPR cannot be performed in the water; the victim must be positioned on a hard surface before the technique is effective.

The possibility of drowning becomes an additional hazard in aquatic exercise that is not found in landbased programs. As an aquatic exercise instructor, it is not mandatory to also be a trained lifeguard; however, it is imperative that you have some basic water safety training. The American Red Cross offers a variety of training programs for persons working in, or around, water settings. It is advisable to have a lifeguard on duty in addition to the exercise instructor (even if the instructor is a certified lifeguard). Some states will require this, while others do not have specific rulings on this situation; for the safety of participants and the liability of the instructor and the facility, it is highly recommended. As an instructor, you should be able to give your full attention to teaching and interacting with participants. If you also are required to become the primary rescuer because there is no lifeguard on duty, your attention becomes divided and your effectiveness to perform either duty decreases. Should an emergency situation arise, the lifeguard can initiate the rescue, while the instructor can clear the pool of class participants and then initiate any other duties described in the emergency action plan. Drowning accidents can occur very quickly; you must be prepared before the situation arises.

REACHING ASSISTS

Some simple techniques the instructor and the participants should be familiar with include reaching and throwing assists. If the person in distress is close to the pool edge, it is often possible to reach that person with your arm or leg, or with a piece of rescue equipment. Most pools will have rescue tubes or buoys, shepherds crooks and/or poles located in conspicuous areas, and you should always familiarize yourself with the location of such equipment. However, if equipment is not available, you also can extend a kickboard, towel, or piece of clothing. When making a reaching assist, you must maintain a position of safety. Keep your center of gravity as low as possible when reaching from the deck, and lean away from the pool's edge if standing on deck.

THROWING ASSISTS

Throwing assists may be required if the distressed person is farther from the pool edge, especially if a shepherds crook or pole is not available. Throwing assists require practice to make them safe and effective. Again the rescuer must maintain a position of safety; one end of the throwing device must remain on deck (stand on the non-throwing end of the rope or secure a loop around your wrist) so that the victim can be pulled to safety; proper aiming and positioning of the device are imperative.

MOUTH-TO-MOUTH BREATHING

Although it was previously stated that CPR cannot be conducted in the pool, mouth-to-mouth breathing techniques can be modified and performed in the water. The rescuer assumes what is termed the "do-si-do" position with the victim; extend your right arm between the victim's right arm and body, positioning your forearm under the back of the victim. (This can be performed from the left side just as easily.) This

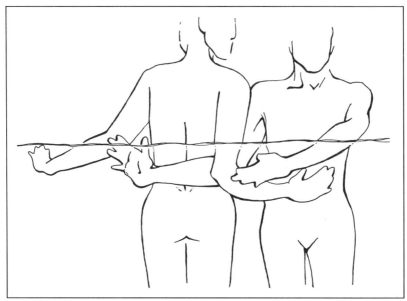
Preparing for the do-si-do position.

will allow you to provide some flotation to the victim and also leave your other arm free to open the airway and pinch the nostrils during the mouth-to-mouth breathing. If you are in shallow water, you can remain standing, and if close to the pool edge, you can hold on to the pool edge with the arm positioned under the victim. If you are in deep water, some type of flotation device will be needed for either yourself or the victim.

Again, if you are not comfortable with any of these techniques you should contact a water safety training organization for further information. Do not wait until an emergency happens - be prepared.

EMERGENCY ACTION PLAN

Each facility should have an emergency action plan which is known and understood by all personnel, including the water exercise instructor and class participants. This will delineate the chain of command and the responsibilities of each individual should an emergency situation occur. According to the American Red Cross, an emergency plan should not only provide proper care of the victim(s), but also address crowd control and supervision of the facility. As every facility will have different procedures and guidelines, it is important to know and understand the emergency plan prior to conducting a class.

CONTRAINDICATIVE EXERCISES

The potential adverse effects of certain movements contraindicates their inclusion in a safe exercise program. Some movements may be suitable for a physical therapy program but not advisable in a multi-level class performed on a repetitive basis. Some movements may be suitable for certain individuals, but not suitable to others due to fitness level or physical limitation. One should always evaluate a movement for potential problems before including it in the class program. Common movements seen in water exercise programs which may be contraindicative include:

Lunges (compromise the knee joint; correction: never allow the front knee to go past a 90-degree angle)

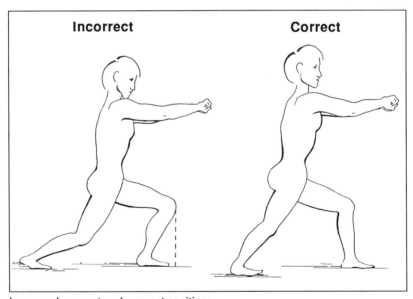

Lunges: Incorrect and correct positions.

Prone Flutterkicks holding to the wall or a kickboard (possible hyperextension of the cervical and/or lumbar vertebrae; correction: keep the head in a neutral position, let the legs remain lower than the shoulders or change to a vertical position in deep water)

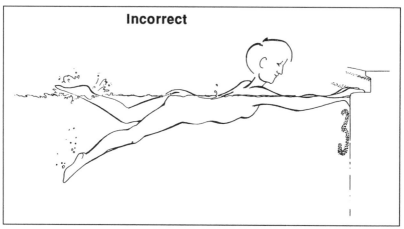

Incorrect position for prone flutterkick; cervical and lumbar vertebrae are hyperextended.

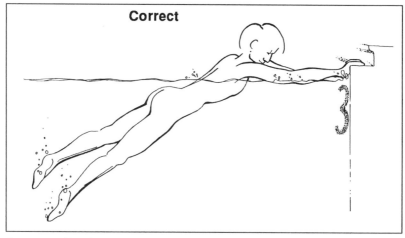

Correct position for prone flutterkick; spine is in a more neutral position.

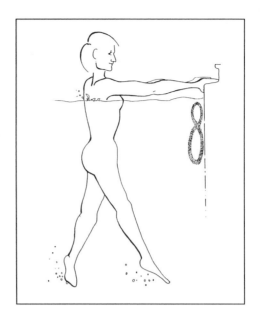

Option for flutterkick -
vertical position.

Back Kicks (possible hyperextension of the lumbar vertebrae;
correction: bring the arm(s) forward of the body as the leg kicks
back and keep the kicks low)

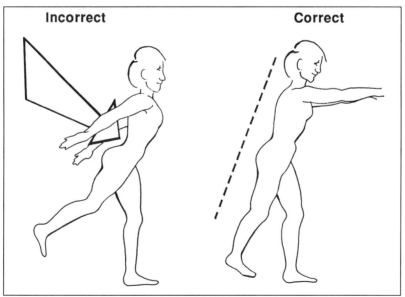

Incorrect   **Correct**

Back kick: Incorrect and correct positions.

Full Neck Circles (hyperextension of the cervical vertebrae; correction: circle the head slowly from shoulder to shoulder - only in front of the body)

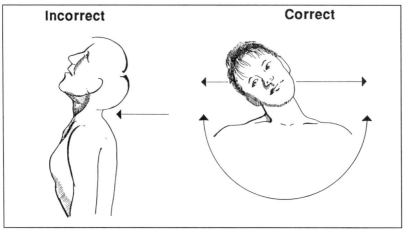

Neck Circles: Incorrect and correct positions.

Twisting (stresses the spine and knee joints; correction: avoid twisting with the feet stationary - the knee and toe of the same foot should always face in the same direction, let the opposite heel lift and turn on the ball of the foot when performing a non-impact twisting motion or let both feet lift from the pool bottom when performing an impact twisting motion; adjust speed and range of motion for each individual)

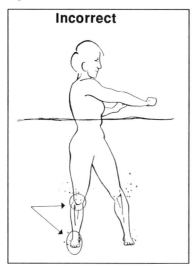

Twisting with feet planted; can stress knee and ankle joints.

Non-impact twisting movement allowing the heel to lift and the body to rotate to protect the knee and ankle joints.

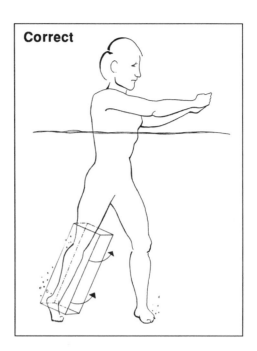

Correct

Impact twisting movement allowing the feet and knees to remain facing the same direction throughout the exercise.

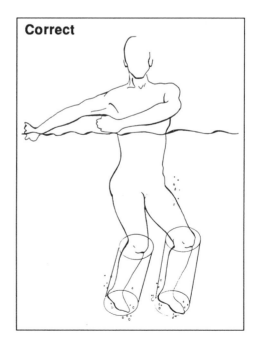

Correct

Wall-Hanging Exercises (shoulder impingement and hyperextension of the lumbar vertebrae; correction: do not perform an excessive number of exercises from this position - change body position or take breaks to ease the stress on the shoulders, or perform the exercises in deep water with a flotation device that does not cause stress to the shoulder joint; be aware of body alignment especially in participants with weak abdominal muscles; realize that some "abdominal" exercises performed from this position are primarily working the hip flexors and opt for a different exercise altogether)

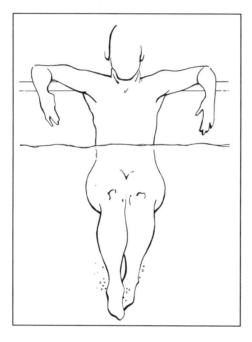

Position for wall hanging exercises - may cause stress to the shoulder lower back.

As we should be well aware, the adage "no pain, no gain" does NOT apply to participants in a fitness class. If an exercise causes pain, do not do that exercise! Even the most basic exercise may not be acceptable for certain individuals.

BODY ALIGNMENT

POSTURAL ANALYSIS

Good posture is an important factor in looking and feeling good, but good posture also is critical in maintaining proper body alignment during exercise. Your mother's simple advice to stand up straight and pull your shoulders back was well worth heeding. Unfortunately, many have forgotten, and our everyday lives cause further deviation by emphasizing movements in front of the body. Take a moment and evaluate your posture; truth be known, most of us would be caught slumped in our chairs or standing with our shoulders rounded!

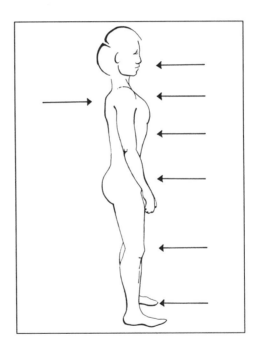

Correct postural alignment.

When standing, one's head should be centered over the shoulders, shoulders over the hips, hips over the knees, and knees over the ankles. The chin should be lifted, the shoulder blades pulled back but relaxed down, the rib cage lifted, the buttocks slightly tucked, and the knees not locked and facing in the same direction as the toes. It is just as important not to overemphasize these positions, as it is not to neglect them. Some individuals will have a physical anomaly which will cause deviations from this alignment - curvatures of the spine (scoliosis, lordosis and kyphosis), inversion or eversion of the feet, or one leg being slightly longer than the other are common problems. However, many postures suffer from muscular imbalance or just lack of body awareness - these can easily be corrected by a well-designed exercise program.

DURING EXERCISE

The exercise program should encourage and develop good posture. During transitions from one movement to another the body may be temporarily out of alignment, but the body should not remain in a compromising position for an extended length of time. Frequent verbal and visual cueing from the instructor will increase body awareness and encourage participants to maintain proper alignment. Participants with good body alignment are less likely to suffer injuries (during class and everyday activities) and also will see better results from the exercise program. An added benefit of good posture is improved breathing techniques, and proper breathing leads to increased abdominal muscle tone.

MUSCLE BALANCE

Muscle balance should be a major goal of any fitness program. Although the water itself provides a better balance by providing resistance in both directions, there are specific guidelines to include. Muscle balance would obviously involve exercising both sides of the body during the same workout, but also would require exercises for both the upper and lower body muscle groups. In addition, it is important to exercise opposing muscle groups during the same workout, for example the biceps and triceps, the hamstrings and quadriceps, the hip abductors and adductors. And, if a muscle is worked, then it also should be properly stretched to prevent a decrease in range of motion. It would be difficult to include specific isolation exercises for every muscle group during a single workout, but be sure to work both the right and left sides, exercise opposing muscles, and stretch what is strengthened. Finally, determine that all muscle groups are properly trained during the overall course outline.

CONCENTRIC vs ECCENTRIC CONTRACTIONS

Muscles are capable of performing different types of contractions - isometric, isotonic, and isokinetic. Isometric exercises involve very little change in the length of the muscle during the contraction; i.e. pushing against an immovable object. This type of contraction allows for strength gains, but only at the angle of the contraction, not through the muscle's full range of motion. Isokinetic contractions would allow for a constant force or speed throughout the range of movement and would be possible only when exercising on specifically designed equipment. Most exercise classes rely on isotonic contractions to strengthen and tone the muscles; there are two types of isotonic contractions - concentric and eccentric.

Concentric contractions occur when the muscle exerts a force that results in muscular torque that is greater than resistance torque; eccentric contractions occur when the muscle exerts a force that results in muscular torque that is less than resistance torque. Concentric contractions involve the shortening of the muscle to move the bone at a joint; eccentric contractions are a lengthening of the muscle (to its original length). Since gravity is a force which pulls all objects toward the earth, in order to lift a weight the muscles must be able to create a force greater than the force of gravity. An example would be a bicep curl on land: hold a dumbbell in one hand with the arm at the side of the body and flex (bend) the elbow joint to bring the dumbbell up in front of the body toward the shoulder - concentric contraction of the biceps; with control, allow the arm to return to the starting position - eccentric contraction of the biceps. Because gravity would pull the arm back down to the starting position in this example, the triceps are not involved as a primary mover because there is no resistance to work against. Gravity causes the movement, but the biceps eccentrically contract to control the speed of that movement. The same principle would apply even if the dumbbell was not held, as the bicep would be working against the force of gravity to flex the elbow and working with gravity to extend (straighten) the elbow.

However, when submerged in water we have previously discussed that buoyancy force cancels out much of the gravitational pull. When exercising in the water then, movements are usually the result of concentric contractions only. Refer back the example of the bicep curl. If the arm is submerged in the water while performing the exercise, a concentric contraction of the bicep flexes (bends) the elbow while a concentric contraction of the tricep extends (straightens) the elbow. This is because the water acts as resistance for movement in both directions, so the tricep will have to shorten (concentric contraction) to move the forearm to an extended position. This principle in itself allows the water medium to provide an exercise program more suited to muscular balance because muscle pairs are always being worked together.

STRENGTHEN AND STRETCH

Progressive overload to the muscular system will cause hypertrophy (growth) of the muscle fibers. Strong muscles are not necessarily injury-free; no matter how strong the muscle, if the range of motion is decreased, the muscle is likely to become injured. A muscle that is not properly stretched becomes "tight" - the muscle fibers remain in a shortened state. Muscular strength is a major component of physical fitness, but flexibility is also, and unfortunately it is often overlooked when participating in an exercise program. (Note: decrease in range of motion can also be a result of trauma within the joint itself such as arthritis, tendonitis, and bursitis.)

A well-designed aquatic program will include a pre-stretch near the beginning of class to prepare the muscles for the workout to follow, and a post-stretch at the end of class to increase flexibility. Therefore, it is important for participants to attend the entire class because arriving late or leaving early can lead to muscle injury.

EVALUATING AN EXERCISE

There is no perfect exercise; any movement can potentially cause injury, but this should not create a fear about leading or participating in a fitness class. Proper education, and learning to understand our own bodies, will help ensure a safe and effective workout. The safety of an exercise or movement depends upon the speed of execution, body alignment and the ability level of the participant.

All movement should be performed at a speed that allows for smooth and controlled performance. Quick, jerking movements often lead to musculo-skeletal injuries and seldom are effective in their intent. As discussed previously, water as an exercise medium requires movements to be slower than when exercising on land. The depth of the water also will affect speed; deeper water will generally require slower movement, provided that body alignment is not compromised.

Any given exercise should allow the participant to maintain proper body alignment throughout its execution. The joints should remain slightly relaxed ("soft") rather than being rigidly locked or hyperextended. Be conscious of working, and stretching, the muscles rather than the tendons and ligaments within the joint. Muscle tissue is elastic and is designed to change length so that movement can occur; however, the tendons and especially the ligaments are less elastic, so overstretching can result in permanent damage.

No two individuals are exactly alike, therefore each participant responds somewhat differently to the same exercise. We have previously discussed ways of modifying intensity levels, but it may be necessary to substitute a completely different exercise in some instances. For example, it is suggested that exercise participants who have had hip replacement surgery not take the leg past the midline of the body. Therefore an exercise that causes one leg to cross in front of the other should be avoided and a different exercise substituted. No one should be encouraged to perform any movement which is uncomfortable.

EVALUATING A PROGRAM

By incorporating all we have discussed in the previous topics on safety, you can easily evaluate the safety of any aquatic exercise program. All the components need to be realized: the facility should meet safety requirements, the instructor should be properly trained, the program should not include contraindicative exercises and modifications for various situations should be provided as the need arises, body alignment should be maintained and encouraged, and the format of the program should promote muscle balance.

Although safety is a primary concern, even the safest class will not be effective if it is not enjoyable simply because people will not continue to participate. In order to provide the results the participants desire, the class format and style must be developed accordingly. In general, do the participants want to socialize or exercise, do they want to develop strength or improve aerobic capacity, do they want to lose body fat or gain flexibility? Answers to questions such as these are important to determine the class structure and the instructor's presentation style. Determining this becomes more complicated when classes must try to meet the needs of various ages, abilities, and desires; at some point, it may become necessary to separate into different class levels and formats so that everyone can, and will, continue to participate.

INSTRUCTOR SAFETY

An aquatic exercise instructor not only has the responsibility of providing a safe environment for the students, but also must be aware of his/her own safety. The instructor becomes a role model for all the participants, and jeopardizing one's health and safety does not provide a good example.

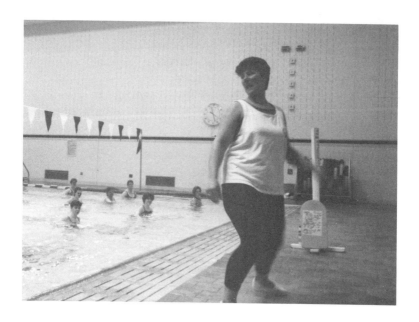

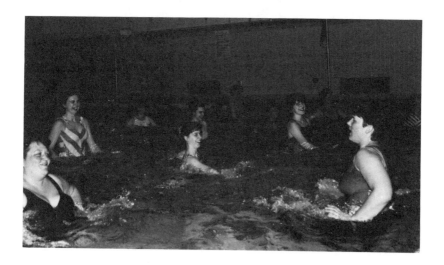

DECK vs WATER

A question of utmost concern is whether the instructor should teach class from the deck or in the water. Actually, a good instructor should have the ability to do both (unless a physical limitation prohibits teaching from one location or the other) because both have their advantages and disadvantages.

Teaching from the deck is beneficial in that students can easily see the instructor and observe correct body alignment. The instructor also can make a better observation of the entire class; when teaching in the pool it is very difficult to see those participants on the back row, especially if the class is large. It is usually easier for the participants to hear the verbal cues when the instructor teaches from deck. Problems arise from the fact that pool decks are generally an unyielding surface, such as concrete, which increases the amount of impact to the body, and because decks often are wet and slippery, creating additional hazards. Also, the instructor is not surrounded by water, it becomes difficult to maintain proper speed — one tends to revert to land speed which is, of course, too fast for the students. The pool environment is typically hot and humid; this is not conducive to vigorous exercise, and the instructor is in danger of heat-related illness.

Certain precautions are important when instructing from the pool edge. Use low impact at all times; the students in the water will be able to jump and bounce, but the instructor on deck should avoid these movements and instead rely on cueing techniques to describe the exercise. To avoid becoming overheated, work at a low intensity, dress appropriately and drink plenty of water. And although performing exercises at land speed is not likely to be a hazard for the instructor, it can become a problem for students trying to follow the exercise. A good instructor will take the time to master the technique of teaching water speed while standing on deck.

There is no doubt that teaching in the water is more comfortable for the instructor, and in many cases more enjoyable for everyone, because better student-teacher interaction can be developed. The instructor also will be able to motivate participants by performing the movements with the same impact and intensity level. There are also a few exercises, such as tuck jumps, wall-hanging exercises and deep water moves, that are virtually impossible to demonstrate from the deck; students need to see them performed in the water to properly understand technique and alignment.

Often beginners understand better when the instructor remains on deck, but as they become accustomed to the program, the instructor can spend more time in the pool. So overall, it is best to use a combination of teaching locations.

VOCAL CORD INJURY

A common health hazard associated with exercise instructors is stress on the vocal cords. This can result from improper breathing and speaking techniques, music that is too loud, and, especially in pool situations, poor acoustics and the presence of chemicals in the air. An instructor should be able to project his/her voice so that students can hear without the need for yelling; a microphone may be required. Music, although motivating, should not be so loud that it inhibits verbal cueing by the instructor. Some instructors utilize music tapes with verbal cues dubbed in; this saves the instructor's voice for motivating and correcting. The chemicals used in the water (such as chlorine and bromine) can create problems for the instructor, from minor irritation to allergic reactions; the chemicals tend to dry out the larynx and trachea, causing additional stress to the vocal cords when talking. Drinking water before, during and after class will be helpful and prevent dehydration.

REFERENCES

The American Red Cross. *Lifeguard Training*. Washington, D.C.: The American Red Cross, 1983 and 1984.

Thompson, Clem W. *Manual of Structural Kinesiology, 11th Edition*. St Louis: Times Mirror/Mosby Publishing, 1989.

The Aquatic Exercise Association Instructor Certification Program, Aquatic Exercise Association, Port Washington, WI.

Howley, Edward T. and Franks, B. Don. *Health/Fitness Instructor's Handbook*. Champaign, IL: Human Kinetics Publishers, Inc., 1986.

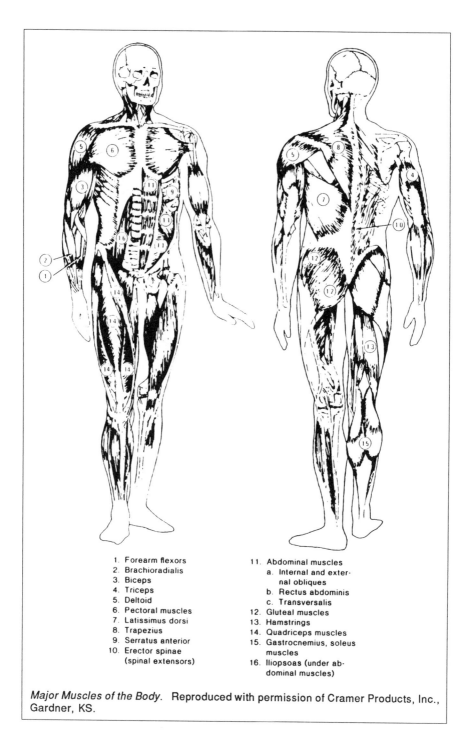

1. Forearm flexors
2. Brachioradialis
3. Biceps
4. Triceps
5. Deltoid
6. Pectoral muscles
7. Latissimus dorsi
8. Trapezius
9. Serratus anterior
10. Erector spinae
    (spinal extensors)
11. Abdominal muscles
    a. Internal and exter-
       nal obliques
    b. Rectus abdominis
    c. Transversalis
12. Gluteal muscles
13. Hamstrings
14. Quadriceps muscles
15. Gastrocnemius, soleus
    muscles
16. Iliopsoas (under ab-
    dominal muscles)

Major Muscles of the Body. Reproduced with permission of Cramer Products, Inc., Gardner, KS.

Chapter 3

CONDUCTING
CLASS

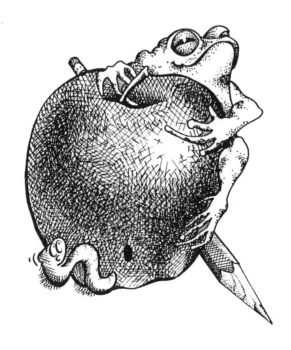

GENERAL CLASS FORMAT

A well designed aquatic aerobic exercise class will basically follow the following format: Muscular/Skeletal Warm-up (Thermal Warm-up), Pre-Stretch, Cardio-Respiratory Warm-up, Cardio-Respiratory Training, Muscle Toning/ Strengthening, and Final Stretch. Although the different phases often overlap, there is a specific purpose for each. The overall focus of the class, the participants' abilities and interests, and the time schedule will determine the specifics, but some general guidelines to follow are listed below.

MUSCULAR/SKELETAL WARM-UP (THERMAL WARM-UP)

Since the suggested water temperature for aquatic aerobic exercise is 80-84 degrees Fahrenheit, and normal body temperature is 98.6 degrees, the water will feel cold when first immersed. Cold muscles are not conducive to stretching or vigorous exercise, so the intent of the thermal warm-up is to elevate the temperature of the muscles through gentle rhythmic movements, beginning with short levers and a small range of motion and gradually developing to long levers and full range of motion. These movements will cause an increased blood flow, and thereby increased oxygen delivery, to the muscles and also will release synovial fluid within the joints which acts as a lubricant to make movement easier.

Typically 3-5 minutes is adequate for the thermal warm-up, but if the water temperature is cooler, as long as 10 minutes may be required for participants to become comfortable. Also, the colder the water, the more vigorous the movements will be needed to appropriately elevate the body temperature.

PRE-STRETCH

At one point, leaders in the fitness industry advocated initiating the workout with stretches, but through research, and participant feedback, it was found that it was not beneficial to stretch "cold" muscles. Therefore, the pre-stretch should follow an adequate thermal warm-up. The intent of the pre-stretch is not to improve flexibility, but rather to prepare the muscles for the exercises to follow. The major muscle groups to be worked should be stretched (holding the stretches for approximately 10 seconds) before the vigorous phase of work is initiated. In a general class setting it is recommended to incorporate static, not ballistic, stretches to provide the safest and most efficient results.

The pre-stretch will last about 3-5 minutes in most class situations and may overlap somewhat with the thermal warm-up, such as intermixing rhythmic limbering movements with static stretches for the same muscle group. Because the water cools the body more effectively than air, the muscles can quickly become cold, inhibiting the ability to stretch safely. One way to prevent this is to continue movement of other body parts while statically stretching a particular muscle. As an example, when performing a static calf-stretch, let the arms continue to swing at the sides to help maintain an elevated body temperature. If the water is below the recommended temperature, caution should be taken during the pre-stretch so that muscles are not injured.

CARDIO-RESPIRATORY WARM-UP

Just as the muscles of the body are prepared to workout, it is necessary to adequately prepare the cardio-respiratory system. The heart rate should be gradually elevated into the working range (target heart rate) and the respiratory system should be gradually overloaded. Similar movements as found in the thermal warm-up are effective, such as jogging, bouncing, and kneelifts, but they now become more vigorous. Once again, most class situations will require approximately 3-5 minutes to accomplish the goals of this warm-up segment.

CARDIO-RESPIRATORY TRAINING

This segment is the main focus of an aquatic aerobic class; the purpose is to improve cardiac output and oxygen delivery. It is imperative that the heart rate be maintained continuously within the target zone for a minimum of 20 minutes to meet the guidelines set forth by ACSM to promote cardio-respiratory fitness and body composition in a healthy adult.

The exact goals and the ability levels of the participants, as well as the length of time allotted, will determine the intensity and duration of the aerobic training portion of class. A typical, one-hour aquatic class will have 20-30 minutes of aerobic activity and will develop a gradual increase/peak/decrease in intensity during that time period. Activities such as walking, jogging, jumping, kicking and leaping provide movements that are aerobic in nature, and by incorporating the methods described in Chapter One, the intensity level can be easily adjusted. Types of programs, and respective variations in the aerobic segment, will be discussed later in this chapter.

Should a major goal of the class be the improvement of participant's body composition (decreasing the percentage of body fat), it is generally recommended to have a long duration, low intensity aerobic segment. During exercise, the human body is always incorporating a combination of carbohydrates and fats as a fuel source; however, the proportion can be manipulated to some degree. High intensity exercise utilizes a greater proportion of carbohydrates, whereas low intensity exercise utilizes a greater proportion of fats. Studies have shown that at 30 minutes of continuous walking, the fuel source is about an equal percentage of carbohydrates and fats; continued exercise past this point will increase the percentage of fat utilized. Two other factors that impact the proportion of fuel metabolized by the body during exercise is the cardio-respiratory fitness level (a more "fit" person is able to utilize a higher percentage of fat) and the dietary intake of the individual.

MUSCLE TONING/STRENGTHENING

The goal of this portion of class is to effectively isolate and strengthen various muscle groups. Remember to promote muscle balance through a well-designed format.

Although the stated goal is necessary to address, this segment is optional because the water provides 12 times the resistance of air, and the resistance is effective in all directions of movement, therefore the muscles of the body are being toned and strengthened even during the aerobic phase of class. Some instructors, and participants, prefer to include a separate segment to isolate specific muscle groups; this is especially effective if additional equipment is incorporated.

Caution should be taken that participants do not become chilled during this segment as injuries could result. Because muscle groups are being isolated during this segment of class, the body temperature will decrease rather quickly, especially if the water or air temperature is lower than recommended. Also recall that fat serves to insulate the body from the cold, so participants who have a low percentage of body fat may chill more easily than others.

An option for the the toning/strengthening segment is to include it at the beginning of class after the pre-stretch has been completed and before the cardio-respiratory warm-up has been initiated.

FINAL STRETCH

Improvement in flexibility is the goal of the final segment of class. This segment is often overlooked by participants and instructors alike, but flexibility is a major component of physical fitness, and like any system of the body, it is susceptible to the principle of reversibility. One must continually train, through gradual progressive overload, the flexibility system of the body to develop improvements in range of motion.

The stretches in this segment should be static and held for about 15-30 seconds. Because the body will become cold while standing for several minutes, it is important to move the limbs that are not being stretched (such as gentle bouncing in place while stretching the upper body). Another option, and one that is advisable if the water temperature is too cold, is to have participants move to deck for the final stretch.

MONITORING INTENSITY

According to the ACSM guidelines, in order for a workout to be considered an aerobic activity, the intensity must fall within the designated parameters: 50-85% of maximum oxygen uptake (VO max), or 50-85% of the heart rate reserve as calculated by the Karvonen Formula, or 60-90% of maximal heart rate. Since it is impractical, if not impossible, for most instructors to gain access to the equipment required to measure VO max, we will discuss the other options for monitoring intensity levels of a workout.

It is important also to note that it is generally accepted that heart rates will be lower when exercising in the water than when exercising on land. Several properties of water are likely factors in this difference: the force of gravity is greatly reduced when submerged in the water, therefore the circulatory system does not have to work as hard to pump blood from the extremities to the heart; water compresses the body, including the circulatory system, and the venous return of blood to the heart is facilitated by this compression; gases (oxygen) enter into a liquid (blood) more readily under pressure so the heart can more easily distribute oxygen to the working muscles; and the water cools the body more efficiently than the air, so the heart does not have to work as hard to dissipate the heat created by exercise.

A study performed at Adelphi University involved 10 female subjects who performed identical dance routines - on land and then again in the water. Oxygen uptake, heart rates, and perceived exertion were measured during both situations. It was found that although the water sequence elicited a 13% lower heart rate, the metabolic data showed a cardio-respiratory training stimulus of approximately 80% of maximal oxygen uptake (VO). It was concluded that although heart rates were lower in aquatic exercise, the metabolic benefits were comparable.

Another study documented by Katch, Katch, and McCardle, 1981, showed similar results in heart rate responses. The conclusion from this study was a 17 beat per minute (bpm) deduction from the training zone when exercising in water. The Aquatic Exercise Association currently utilizes this deduction to arrive at an aquatic heart rate modification.

If heart rates are to be utilized when determining intensity levels in aquatic exercise, it is suggested that a six-second pulse count be taken because the heart rate will return more quickly to the pre-exercise rate than when exercising on land. Always use one or two fingertips to monitor pulse (not the thumb); the pulse may be felt at the carotid artery at the side of the neck or the radial artery at the wrist.

KARVONEN FORMULA

The Karvonen Formula utilizes the individual's age and resting heart rate (the number of times the heart beats per minute while at rest) to determine the training zone for that person. The resting heart rate is included in the calculation to make the formula more individualized; it is generally found that as a person obtains a higher level of cardio-respiratory fitness, his or her resting heart rate will decrease.

Step One: 220 - Age of Individual = Maximal Heart Rate

Step Two: Maximal HR - Resting HR = HR Reserve

Step Three:
HR Reserve x 0.50 = 50% of HR Reserve
HR Reserve x 0.85 = 85% of HR Reserve

Step Four:
50% of HR Reserve + Resting HR = Minimum Working HR
                                        (Land-based exercise)

85%of HR Reserve + Resting HR = Maximum Working HR
                                        (Land-based exercise)

Step Five:
Minimum Working HR - 17 bpm = Minimum Working HR
(Land-based exercise)   (Aquatic exercise)

Maximum Working HR - 17 bpm = Maximum Working HR
(Land-based exercise)   (Aquatic exercise)

The target zone, or training zone, is between the minimum and maximum working heart rate as determined by the formula. In order for the workout to be considered aerobic in nature, the heart rate must remain within this range for a minimum of 20 minutes continuously.

MAXIMAL HEART RATE FORMULA

An alternate method for determining target heart rate ranges is the Maximum Heart Rate Formula; this is very similar to the Karvonen Formula but does not take into consideration the individual's resting heart rate. The M.H.F. is based strictly on the age, not the fitness level, of the participant. Many class situations utilize this method because the target zones can be calculated for age groups, and posted for quick reference by participants. With the Maximal Heart Rate Formula, ACSM allows for the target zone of 60-90%.

Step One: 220 - Age = Maximal Heart Rate

Step Two:
Maximal HR x 0.60 = Minimum Working HR (Land-based exercise)
Maximal HR x 0.90 = Maximum Working HR (Land-based exercise)

Step Three:
Minimum Working HR - 17 bpm = Minimum Working HR
(Land-based exercise)   (Aquatic exercise)

Maximum Working HR - 17 bpm= Maximum Working HR
(Land-based exercise)   (Aquatic exercise)

The target zone, or training zone, is between the minimum and maximum working heart rate as determined by the formula. In order for the workout to be considered aerobic in nature, the heart rate must remain within this range for a minimum of 20 minutes continuously.

PERCEIVED EXERTION

The Rating of Perceived Exertion (RPE), as a method of determining intensity levels of exercise, was developed by Borg. His studies concluded that heart rates and verbal descriptions of participant's perceived activity levels were closely correlated; when a person feels that he or she is working "somewhat hard" to "hard", they are usually within their target heart rate range (original rating scale).

Utilizing perceived exertion to monitor intensity levels causes the participant to pay close attention to his or her specific response to exercise. Many factors, besides the exercise program, will impact the heart rate: medication (prescription drugs as well as "over the counter" medications, alcohol, caffeine and nicotine), environmental conditions, and type of clothing can create variations in heart rate response.

Another problem eliminated by perceived exertion is that many individuals are unable to accurately monitor their own heart rate. To be accurate, the pulse must be counted immediately after the exercise segment is completed; it is suggested that the participant keep moving while the pulse is counted. This can be difficult, if not impossible, for some participants to master. The problem may be compounded in aquatic exercise because heart rates drop more quickly after the exercise is terminated, and the movement of water on the body often makes it more difficult to actually count the pulse. On the other hand, most everyone in a class situation can accurately describe how they feel during any given exercise.

TALK TEST

A somewhat less scientific method of intensity monitoring is referred to as the "Talk Test". Talking is a secondary response of the respiratory system, so if a participant is unable to answer a simple question during an exercise segment because he or she requires full attention to supplying oxygen to the body (breathing), the intensity level is most likely too high. In other words, the person is probably working over his or her maximum target heart rate range at that point.

This method does not provide for monitoring the full target heart rate zone, but merely indicates that the maximum intensity has been exceeded.

RESPIRATION RATE

The respiration rate (number of breaths per minute) shows a noticeable increase when an individual approaches his or her minimum aerobic intensity level because aerobic activity requires oxygen to generate sufficient ATP (adenosine tri-phosphate) to meet energy demands. Whereas the "Talk Test" indicates that the maximum intensity level has been exceeded, an increase in respiration rate will indicate that the minimum intensity level has been reached.

In simple terms, if during the aerobic segment of class an individual is still breathing at a pre-exercise rate, that person is not working at a sufficient level to provide cardio-respiratory training.

TYPES OF PROGRAMS

Aquatic programs can be designed around most any class format found in land-based exercise. Classes are being offered in circuit training, interval training, sports specific programs, water walking/water jogging, deep water exercise, aqua benching, aqua power, and non-aerobic toning to name a few. Program formats also can be geared toward special population groups such as older adults, pre- and post-natal women, children, athletes, and the physically impaired. Water provides an environment that can be challenging, yet not stressful, and with minor modifications in formatting the program can suit most any need.

CIRCUIT TRAINING

Circuit training is generally considered to consist of a program that alternates between aerobic activities and strengthening/toning activities. The goal is to keep participants moving constantly between each activity station, and by intermixing aerobic-type exercises with the muscle conditioning exercises, the heart rate may be maintained within the target heart rate range.

Two methods of instruction are individual and group travel. Group travel is somewhat easier for the instructor to monitor, as the class moves from station to station as one unit, and instructions and cautions need be explained only once for each exercise. The possible drawback to this method is that if equipment is being utilized, there must be an adequate supply for everyone. The other method allows for the class to divide into as many sub-groups as there are stations; when the signal is given each sub-group will move to the next station and initiate the new exercise. This makes it more difficult for the instructor, as he or she will have to monitor all exercise stations continually to provide information and motivation for each sub-group. It will be helpful to have each exercise clearly explained in writing, and/or diagrams, at every station so that sub-groups will have a constant reference. One benefit to this method is that many different types of equipment can be utilized without the need to provide for every class participant; if the maximum number in each sub-group is three, then only three pieces, or sets, of each type of equipment is required. This allows for great variety, and yet remains cost-effective.

The class follows the basic guidelines described in GENERAL CLASS FORMAT, described on page 38, except that the muscle toning/strengthening segment is interspersed within the cardio-respiratory training segment. All ability levels can effectively work together in this type of class; the instructor should motivate participants to work with adequate intensity to maintain their heart rates within the target zone.

Listed below is a sample circuit of eight basic stations and the focus of each exercise; emphasis is on lower body and torso movements only for simplicity. To provide adequate upper body strengthening and toning, incorporate strict arm movements in conjunction with the exercises listed, or additional stations for specific upper body muscles. Although equipment is optional, it will provide greater gains in strength and muscle tone.

Station 1	Pendulum (rock side)	Aerobic
Station 2	Side leg lift and cross over	Strength - inner and outer thighs
Station 3	Jumping Jacks	Aerobic
Station 4	Knee extension/flexion	Strength - quads and hamstrings
Station 5	Kicks -front, side, and back	Aerobic
Station 6	Straight leg swing	Strength - buttocks and hip flexors
Station 7	Twisting with bounce	Aerobic
Station 8	Water pulls	Strength - obliques

INTERVAL TRAINING

Originally developed for individuals in track and field, interval training allowed the athlete to increase the amount of time actually performing at competitive levels for his or her event. Interval training involves work cycles consisting of a high intensity exercise period and a recovery period (usually an "active" rest period of low intensity). This type of training can either be aerobic or anaerobic in nature, and work cycles are developed accordingly.

We will discuss only aerobic interval training; the high intensity (80-85%) aerobic interval would be followed by a low intensity (60-70%) aerobic interval - together these comprise a single work cycle. The heart rate will fluctuate throughout the workout between the minimum and maximum levels, but should remain within the target zone during the entire cardio-respiratory segment. In land-based exercise, aerobic interval training would typically consist of 1:1 ratio of high intensity to low intensity intervals (an equal amount of time spent on each during the work cycle). This ratio should allow participants adequate recovery time after working at near maximum intensity. In aquatic classes, the heart rate will show a faster "recovery" when the intensity level is decreased, and therefore the work ratio may be altered accordingly, possibly a 2:1 (high intensity: low intensity) ratio.

Interval training classes would incorporate the same basic guidelines as listed in the GENERAL CLASS FORMAT; the only necessary modification is in structuring the cardio-respiratory segment around work cycles instead of a gradual increase, peak, and decrease in intensity levels.

Interval training requires a great deal of motivation, both from the instructor and the participants, and is better suited to a more advanced class. However, modifications in work cycle ratios and the intensity levels will allow for any ability level, including multi-level classes, to perform interval training.

A few examples of work cycles are given below; be sure to adjust intensity and impact to suit the participants individuals needs.

Low Intensity	Water walking
High Intensity	"Climb the Wall"
Low Intensity	Lateral travel - step apart then together
High Intensity	Straddle jump on the wall
Low Intensity	Power squat
High Intensity	Straight jump
Low Intensity	Jumping jack
High Intensity	Tuck jump

SPORTS SPECIFIC

Water exercise is being utilized more and more by professional athletes, not only for rehabilitation after injury or surgery, but also as a form of cross training and pre-season preparation. Sports specific water workouts are not limited to professional teams; non-professional and "arm-chair" athletes will benefit as well. Such classes can be geared toward training for a specific sport with special attention on strengthening and stretching various muscle groups to enhance performance. The nature of the sport itself, whether aerobic or non-aerobic, will determine the most effective class format. Some considerations in designing such a program are addressed in the example for softball/ baseball given below.

Softball/Baseball

Common Injuries (see page 36 for diagram of human body)

Shoulder Joint - The shoulder joint is a frequently injured area of the body. The muscular strength of this joint is generally weak and the ligament structure is not strong enough to maintain adequate protection for the joint. The muscles involved are: deltoideus, rotator cuff (supraspinatus, infraspinatus, teres minor, subscapularis), teres major, latissimus dorsi, pectoralis major.

Hamstring - The semitendinosus, semimembranosus, and the biceps femoris muscles are known as the hamstrings. Injuries to this muscle group are common in many sports. The hamstrings often need to be strengthened and stretched to help alleviate injuries.

Muscles to Strengthen

All of the Shoulder Joint Muscles - the rotator cuff muscles and the pectoralis major are strongly involved in throwing movements.

Serratus Anterior Muscle - works along with the pectoralis major in typical action such as throwing a baseball.

Triceps Brachii - the action of the triceps is extension of the elbow and assistance in extension of the shoulder joint; elbow extension is important for a strong swing as well as a strong throwing movement.

Wrist, Hand and Fingers - most sports require strong hands for top performance; daily practice for the sport will often improve skill but not necessarily develop strength.

Legs - all of the muscles of the legs need to be developed as baseball will involve movements in various directions - forward running toward base, lateral movement when preparing to "steal", backwards when watching for a fly ball, etc; important to develop power and speed.

Abdominal Muscles - by strengthening the abdominal muscles (rectus abdominus, internal and external obliques, transversus abdominus) the posture is improved helping to maintain proper body alignment; also the abdominal muscles are involved in forward and lateral flexion and rotation of the trunk - such movements as involved in pitching, batting, bending down to pick up a ground ball, etc.

Stretching

Most baseball/ softball players will benefit from an overall flexibility program with emphasis on the shoulder joint/shoulder girdle, triceps, quadriceps, hip flexors, and hamstrings. Teaching a proper warm-up and stretch routine will encourage participants to utilize this prior to and following the sports event.

Cardio-Respiratory Training

Baseball/softball is not an aerobic sport in that it involves bursts of speed and energy rather than a sustained level of activity, but cardio-respiratory training is still important. Having a strong heart and lungs is beneficial to any person, athlete or not. However, you may want to utilize an interval training format which will allow you to alternate from low intensity to high intensity which would simulate the activity of the sport. Also, you might incorporate some speed drill such as sprints across the pool and some plyometric type moves such as jumps up out of the water — this will help develop necessary skills for the sport (running to base and jumping for a catch).

Another option would be to design a class incorporating sports-oriented moves, rather than moves that are dance-oriented. This type of class may encourage more men to participate in aquatic exercise and will help to develop strength, endurance, and coordination skills necessary to participate in many sports activities.

Basketball Drill

Start with participants in two lines, each pair - the two people across from each other in the lines -will have a ball (i.e. soft child's ball about the size of a basketball).

1. Both people of the pair will travel the same direction on the jog (the passer will be behind the receiver), the receiver only will turn (180 degrees) on counts 5 and 6 to face the passer and catch (hopefully) the ball on counts 7 and 8; the direction of travel will now be reversed and the drill continues.
2. Turn so partners now face each other in the lines, the pair at the "head" of the line will lead down between the lines with a sliding movement and at the same time will alternately throw the ball to each other with a low pass, the remainder will follow with a sliding movement in the opposite direction towards the "head" of the line (to make this more advanced, at the same time these pairs will alternately throw the ball to each other with a high pass); when the first pair gets to the end, they return to the original lines and reverse direction of the slide to move up to the "head" and the drill continues.

Karate Heel Kick

Turn the body toward the right side and kick the left leg forward leading with the heel of the foot (side of leg will be towards the surface of the water); step with the left, right, left turning the body towards the left side and repeat the kick with the right leg.

Soccer Kick

Traveling forward, kick across the body with the arch of the foot as if kicking a soccer ball, then jog 3 times to change legs.

Karate Punch Combo

Lunge to the left side and punch the right arm across the body, return to the center position and punch forward with the left arm; repeat this sequence three more times for a total of 4 sets.

Facing front in a squat stance, punch forward 7 more times and pause on the 8th one with both hands at waist—this will allow you to change sides.

Lunge to the right side and punch the left arm across the body, return to the center position and punch forward with the right arm; repeat this for a total of 4 sets.

Relays and Games

Relays across the pool, or from end to end, are good ways to incorporate traveling steps and drills associated with sports, plus they bring in the feel of competition which most sports enthusiasts enjoy; be sure that team members waiting for their turn keep moving in place.

There are many games on the market (look at your local supplier for home pools) such as floating basketball hoops, volleyball nets for the pool, submerged rings, etc which can easily be incorporated into your aquatics program and will provide variety and fun for you participants.

Any sports-related aquatic workout would still follow the basic guidelines described in GENERAL CLASS FORMAT. Modifications would arise mostly in movement style and intensity levels; sports classes are well suited for use of additional equipment.

WATER WALKING/JOGGING

Shallow water walking classes provide a program that is suitable to many needs, is very low impact as it does not incorporate bouncing, does not require specialized equipment, is effective with or without music accompaniment, and allows for participant interaction as the transition from step to step does not have to be rigidly structured. Water depth can vary from waist to chest deep with participants either moving continually through one depth or traveling from one depth to another to alter the resistance of the workout. To adequately tone and

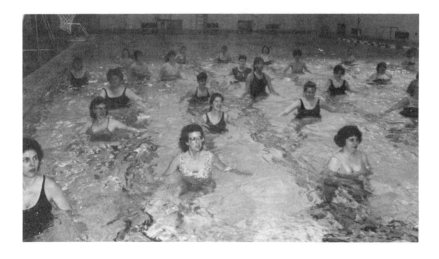

strengthen all of the major muscle groups, the instructor should incorporate a variety of arm and leg movements, change the direction of travel, and utilize both fast and slow speeds throughout the class. Depending upon the size of class and the pool design, participants can travel in one or more circles, in lines across the width of the pool, follow the lane lines as in lap swimming, or any variety of patterns the instructor should choose.

Some examples of steps that could be easily incorporated into a shallow water walking class are listed below; remember to include specific arm movements to tone the muscles of the upper body as well.

Walking with toes forward, pointing out, or pointing in
Large strides - leading with the heel (lead with toe traveling backward)
Tiny steps on the toes or the heels
Step and kneelift with knees lifting across, front or to corner
Step and kick with kicks across, forward or to corner
Walking with heels lifting towards buttocks
Lateral travel with wide steps
Lateral travel with crossing steps

Shallow water jogging is similar to shallow water walking, but the impact is slightly greater in that bouncing type steps are incorporated, and therefore, the intensity is usually increased as well (although water walking can be very intense - for example power striding with impeding arms). A multi-level class might utilize both water walking and jogging steps, allowing participants to make adjustments as needed. Some examples of exercises one might include in a shallow water jogging class are as follows:

Jogs with knees high in front, across, or to corners
Jogs with heels high behind
Traveling Jumping Jacks (less stressful to knees to travel backwards)
Bounces on one or both feet (vary distance between feet)
Leaps forward or lateral
Rocking forward and backward while traveling forward
Rocking side to side (pendulum swing) while traveling laterally
Sliding
Front kicks
Back kicks

In shallow water walking or jogging it is still important to follow the guidelines listed in GENERAL CLASS FORMAT (page 38) to assure a safe and effective program.

DEEP WATER

Deep water programs can be conducted with many different styles; all of the class programs previously discussed - circuit training, interval training, sports specific, and water jogging - can be performed in deep water. Deep water programs are also suitable for any special population that benefits from a non-impact workout, such as pre-natal, post-surgery patients, and obese individuals. Programs conducted in deep water would follow the same GENERAL CLASS FORMAT (page 38) described previously.

Deep water classes do require the use of some type of equipment for flotation. Short periods of deep water exercise might be accomplished without equipment if the participants are physically strong enough to either tread water or scull with the hands to maintain afloat; however, the types of exercises that can be conducted at the same time would be very limited. Buoyancy equipment can be hand-held, attached to the ankles, or fitted around the torso (such as a belt or vest); some equipment provides added resistance as well, but buoyancy is the necessary factor.

In deep water aerobic exercise, the body will typically remain in a vertical position - just as it would in shallow water programs - while leg movements such as marching, jogging, striding, and scissoring are performed to elevate the heart rate into the working range. It is important to emphasize correct posture and body alignment. Persons unaccustomed to exercising in deep water, where their feet do not contact the pool bottom, will benefit from good cueing and demonstration from the instructor. Many people will tend to lean their bodies forward instead of remaining in an upright position; some types of flotation equipment can accenturate this improper body alignment, so choose your equipment carefully.

Exercises can be performed also in a supine position with the aid of the flotation equipment. This is especially beneficial when attempting to isolate and strengthen the abdominal muscles. Each participant should be taught how to safely return to vertical alignment from a supine (or prone) position; this will depend upon the type of equipment being utilized.

Some sample deep water aerobic movements that can be performed are listed on page 54; remember to vary the arm movements depending upon the goal. Arm movements can provide stabilization to maintain body alignment, assistance to travel through the water, or resistance to increase intensity.

Jog with knees high, stationary or traveling forward and backward
Jog with heels high, stationary or traveling forward and backward
Jumping jacks
Scissors (one leg swings forward, one leg swings back)
Striding
Ankle touch, to front or to back

AQUA BENCHING

One of the newest fitness trends is bench stepping, or step aerobics, and we are now seeing a variation being taken into the pool. This type of aquatic program, which requires the use of specialized equipment, involves stepping up and down on a submerged platform or bench (four inches to 12 inches in height) during the aerobic segment of class. This is a relatively new concept for exercise, especially in the water, (although the principle has been utilized for many years in fitness testing), and the instructor would benefit from participating in a specialized, aqua-bench training program. This would provide in-depth information on safety considerations, equipment selection, and specialized choreography.

Proper body alignment, in particular foot placement and knee positioning, is critical to ensure a safe and effective program. One current problem is that the force of the water created during exercise can cause the bench (more suited to land exercise) to move; as the research continues, we will likely see the introduction of a bench specifically designed for the aquatic environment.

AQUA POWER AEROBICS

Aqua power aerobic programs utilize strong, precise moves such as squats and lunges to provide body sculpting during the aerobic portion of class, thus eliminating the need for a separate toning segment (unless a specific abdominal segment is included). The "power moves" are very low impact and suited for all ability levels; it is important for each movement to be controlled and precise to provide the desired goals. By interspersing the "power moves" with other higher intensity moves (such as jog, leaps, jumping jacks, and cross-country skiing), the individual's heart rate can be maintained within the target zone. The overall effect then is a moderate intensity aerobic workout that can be maintained continuously for 45 minutes to an hour and at the same time provide adequate toning and strengthening to the major muscle groups. As discussed in the GENERAL CLASS FORMAT (page 38), if a goal of the participant is to reduce body fat, then the class format should be designed for a long duration aerobic segment. Aqua power aerobics therefore can be beneficial to those desiring to improve their body composition.

The "power moves" can be considered aerobic in that they utilize the large muscle groups of the body in a rhythmic nature, and if performed with adequate exertion they will elevate the heart rate into the lower end of the target zone; they are also strength-oriented because the speed of execution is slower, and the style is precise and controlled, thus allowing a concentrated effort in specific muscle recruitment. This type of class therefore borrows components from both circuit and interval training; the format alternates between high intensity aerobic exercises and "power moves" (low intensity aerobic and strength moves).

The "power moves" are best performed in shallower water, approximately waist to rib-cage deep, so that full range of motion can be obtained. But if the "power moves" are being interspersed with other higher impact and traveling type movements, then deeper water will be suitable; range of motion will be slightly compromised for the sake of increased intensity levels. If the pool design is such that one has access to a range of depths, for example 3 to 5 foot, then the program can be formatted utilizing the entire pool area. The high intensity aerobic segments would be conducted at about chest depth; the "power moves" emphasizing lower body strengthening would be conducted at about waist to rib-cage depth, and finally exercises emphasizing upper body strengthening would be conducted at shoulder depth so that the arms are completely submerged for maximum resistance. Traveling between various locations also will increase the intensity level of the workout.

Other options exist for incorporating "power moves" into an aquatic exercise program besides aerobic training. Since the movements are lower impact and lower intensity, they are ideal for cardio-respiratory warmup and cooldown. The "power moves" can be utilized strictly for toning; because they can be performed in the center of the pool rather than along the edge (where standard toning exercises are generally executed), they will provide variety, encourage better balance and coordination, and help participants to stay warm. An additional benefit to utilizing "power moves" in an aquatic exercise program is that they are similar to movements found in many sports, and therefore may be useful in encouraging male participation.

The class will be designed following the guidelines discussed in GENERAL CLASS FORMAT (page 38), with toning exercises included within the cardio-respiratory segment. Some sample "power moves" are given along with tips on proper body alignment.

Power Squat - the basic move from which many other exercises originate; the feet are in parallel position - knees and toes facing forward with feet about shoulder width apart; the weight of the body is centered over the heels; the abdominals are pulled towards the spine and the lower back is prevented from hyperextending; visualize sitting down into a chair positioned behind you - the knees do not come forward of the ankles; full range of motion would take the knees to a 90-degree angle.

Squat/Side Leg Lift - lifting from the power squat position, one leg is lifted to the side (abduction of the hip); keep the knee and toe of the leg facing toward the front with the knee slightly flexed; return to the power squat and then lift the opposite leg

Squat/ Leg Cross Front - lifting from the power squat position, one leg is lifted across the front toward the opposite side of the body; the hip is rotated outward as the leg lifts; keep the knee slightly flexed; return to the power squat and then lift the opposite leg.

Squat/Hamstring Curl - lifting from the power squat position, bring one heel up behind the body towards the buttock; be careful not to arch the lower back; return to the power squat and then lift the opposite leg.

Squat/Knee Extension - lifting from the power squat position, bring one leg up in front of the body; alternately bend and straighten the leg for a total of 4 or 8 counts; return to the power squat and then lift the opposite leg and repeat

Lunge, Forward - step forward on one leg; keeping the body perpendicular to the pool bottom, bend the knees and lower the body; be careful that the front knee does not extend past the ankle; return to the starting position and step forward with the opposite leg

Lunge, Back - similar to the forward lunge, but the leg steps behind the body to execute the move; some participants find this to be less stressful to the knee joint

AQUA DANCE AEROBICS

In this type of aquatic aerobic exercise, the GENERAL CLASS FORMAT is once again followed. The distinguishing feature is the degree of choreography incorporated into the program. Choreography is simply the arrangement or written notation of movement, and in dance aerobics the choreography should be well planned and rehearsed so that the routines flow smoothly. Some instructors will utilize a completely choreographed "dance" routine for each specific song (as in the example given), where other instructors will sequentially develop a pattern as they teach allowing more freedom in variation of steps.

The movements in this class format are dance-oriented and the sequencing more complex than other types of programs. Movements from all different styles of dance can be incorporated - jazz, funk, ballet, folk - to create unique, and enjoyable, routines. Obviously, music is important to develop style of movement and for motivation; choose music enjoyed by class participants and choreograph the movements accordingly.

Aquatic dance classes will likely attract more women than men. But dance aerobic participants often claim that they have so much fun that they forget they are exercising, so don't be afraid to include this type of class into your schedule. Because of the more complex patterns and steps, coordination and agility can be developed. Be sure to design the choreography to fit the abilities of the participants; if the routine is too complex, they will spend more time "thinking" and less time"working" and thus limit the effectiveness of the workout. The cardio-respiratory warm-up and cool-down offer an ideal time to teach new routines or patterns, as the intensity level is decreased when participants are learning the new moves.

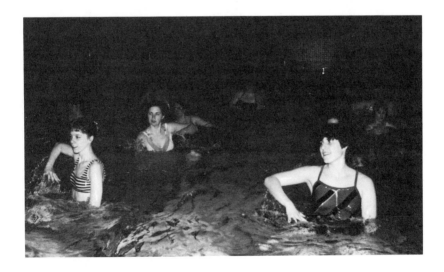

Next is a sample choreographed routine for aquatic exercise.

GIVE ME ONE MORE CHANCE
Music by The Exiles
Choreography by Julie See

Wait 8c

A. Jog 8c - jog to your right in small circle

B. Jog/ Jump
Jog 8c up - lifting heels behind
Jump 4x - as high out of water as possible
Jog 8c back/ Jump 4x
Insert Pause 2c

C. Rock
Face to right and rock slowly 4x (R up, L back, R,L)
Fast 8x - kicking and turning on the 8th one to face left
Repeat to left 4x slowly, 8x fast - end facing front

D. Jog in 3 —Country Style
Jog in 3, adding a flick kick on the fourth count —
knees are lifted out to the side and both arms press
down in front; do 8 sets

Repeat: B, C, D

Repeat: B four times always moving forward with the jogs,
but turning 1/4 turn to right each time to make box pattern

Repeat: A except Jog l0c, then jump apart

Note: Persons requiring a lower impact class can modify the routine by
lifting up to the toes instead of jumping in pattern B.

PERINATAL

Exercise programming for pregnant and postpartum women is another highly specialized field, and it is suggested that instructors participate in a perinatal certification prior to leading such a class on their own. An excellent certification program for aquatic exercise instructors is presented by Barbara Horstmeyer, the Executive Director and Founder of Maternity Fitness, Inc. The basic text for this certification program, which includes both a written and practical test, follows the 1985 guidelines on exercise and pregnancy established by the American College of Obstetricians and Gynecologists (ACOG). These guidelines for exercise during pregnancy and postpartum are based on the unique physical and physiological conditions that exist during these periods. They outline the general criteria for safety to provide direction to patients when developing home exercise programs (land based exercise). The guidelines are listed below.

Pregnancy and Postpartum

1. Regular exercise (at least 3 times per week) is preferable to intermittent activity. Competitive activities should be discouraged.
2. Vigorous exercise should not be performed in hot, humid weather or during a period of febrile illness.
3. Ballistic movements (jerky, bouncy motions) should be avoided. Exercise should be done on a wooden floor or a tightly carpeted surface to reduce shock and provide a sure footing.
4. Deep flexion or extension of joints should be avoided because of connective tissue laxity. Activities that require jumping, jarring motions, or rapid changes in direction should be avoided because of joint instability.
5. Vigorous exercise should be preceded by a 5-minute period of muscle warm-up. This can be accomplished by slow walking or stationary cycling with low resistance.
6. Vigorous exercise should be followed by a period of gradually declining activity that includes gentle stationary stretching. Because connective tissue laxity increases the risk of joint injury, stretches should to be taken to the point of maximum resistance.
7. Heart rate should be measured at times of peak activity. Target heart rates and limits established in consultation with the physician should not be exceeded.

8. Care should be taken to gradually rise from the floor to avoid orthostatic hypotension. Some form of activity involving the legs should be continued for a brief period.
9. Liquids should be taken liberally before and after exercise to prevent dehydration. If necessary, activity should be interrupted to replenish fluids.
10. Women who have led sedentary lifestyles should begin with physical activity of very low intensity and advance activity levels very gradually.
11. Activity should be stopped and the physician consulted if any unusual symptoms appear.

Pregnancy Only

1. Maternal heart rate should not exceed 140 beats per minute.
2. Strenuous activity should not exceed 15 minutes in duration.
3. No exercise should be performed in the supine position after the fourth month of gestation is completed.
4. Exercises that employ the Valsalva maneuver should be avoided.
5. Caloric intake should be adequate to meet not only the extra energy needs of pregnancy, but also of the exercise performed.
6. Maternal core temperature should not exceed 38 degrees C.

Maternity Fitness, Inc. lists some additional guidelines and concerns for aquatic pre-natal exercise.

1. Utilizing the 17 bpm aquatic heart rate deduction would limit the maximal heart rate to 123 bpm rather than 140 bpm.
2. Women must have prior approval from their caregiver to participate in the pre-natal class.
3. Uterine contractions following mild to moderate exercise are common; however, if they occur at regular intervals for more than one hour, the physician should be consulted.
4. Pool temperature should be between 80-83 degrees Fahrenheit; do not attempt to exercise in a therapeutic pool where temperatures are approximately 90 degrees. The maternal core temperature should not exceed the recommended 38 degrees Celciu. *Avoid hot tubs, jacuzzis and whirlpools during pregnancy.*

5. In case of emergency, the phone numbers of the woman's husband and physician, along with the estimated date of confinement, should be immediately available.

A perinatal aquatic exercise class would follow closely with the GENERAL CLASS FORMAT (page 38) previously given, with modifications in the intensity (maximum heart rate not to exceed 123 bpm) and the length of the cardio-respiratory segment (not to exceed 15 minutes). Most exercises and stretches performed in general population class can be utilized. Avoid movements that can cause lower back hyperextension - such as bilateral leg lifts - because of the already increased lordosis and strain to the lower back muscles which often occur during pregnancy.

NON-AEROBIC TONING

Aquatic exercise classes also can be designed to specifically address muscular strength and endurance. Because the program would not include a cardio-respiratory training segment, improvements in aerobic capacity and body composition will not be realized. The class format would begin with a thermal warm-up and pre-stretch, followed by muscular strength and endurance exercises. Sustained stretching is a necessary component to develop and maintain flexibility; each muscle group can be stretched immediately after that specific toning exercise, or an overall, final stretch segment can be included at the end of class.

A toning class is well suited for the use of additional resistance equipment. This would allow for continued, progressive overload of the muscles and provide variety to the workout, both of which will encourage adherence to the program. Participants want to see results and to enjoy the workout - if an instructor can satisfy these goals, students will continue to return to class.

A toning class will be less vigorous than a typical aerobic program; therefore, it might be appealing to the less-conditioned individual. By developing muscular strength and endurance first through a low-intensity toning workout, beginners may later be able to participate in a more strenuous aerobic program without becoming discouraged. This class format is also suitable for a method of cross-training for more physically fit participants; remember that variability in exercise improves training results, overcomes plateaus, and prevents burn-out.

One problem that may occur in a class oriented to toning exercises is that the less vigorous movements may cause participants to become cold. For safety reasons it is important that body temperature remain elevated to a comfortable level. If the pool temperature is warmer than the recommended 80-84 degrees Fahrenheit, the students may be comfortable. Otherwise, encourage participants to dress appropriately (such as a long sleeve, full length unitard rather than a swimsuit) and intersperse more vigorous movements periodically.

Toning exercises can be performed in shallow to deep water and can be conducted from a standing position (in the center of the pool or at the pool edge for support), from a hanging position (in the center of the pool utilizing flotation equipment or with shoulders or hands supporting the body at the pool edge), or from a supine or prone position (utilizing flotation equipment or the wall for support).

BENEFITS

GENERAL HEALTH AND FITNESS

Regular, aquatic aerobic exercise provides a method of improving the five major components of physical fitness (muscular strength, muscular endurance, cardio-respiratory training, flexibility, and body composition) which is safe, effective, and adaptable to most any clientele. Programs can be designed to fit the needs of rehabilitative patients as well as professional athletes, senior citizens as well as children, special populations as well as the general population of exercisers.

If that were not enough, aquatic exercise (and truly most any form of exercise) improves more than just the physical ability and appearance. Regular aquatic exercise can help to develop self esteem, confidence, and camaraderie among participants and instructors. The pool creates an atmosphere that helps to eliminate self-consciousness during exercise - there are no mirrors on the wall and bodies are submerged up to the chest or shoulders so no one else (except an observant instructor) sees that each step is not quite perfect. Water often is the only environment for some individuals where pain-free movement can occur or where they can perform movements that now elude them on land. Aqua exercise can provide an exhilarating workout and then follow up with a soothing, relaxing cool-down. Maybe most important of all is to develop a lifelong "habit" of exercise. Aquatic programs are fun and enjoyable - it seems the water brings out the youth in all its participants.

PERINATAL

The water offers a comfortable environment for most pre-natal and postpartum women. The very properties of water provide improved circulation, less stress to the joints, and greater ease of movement.

Because the effect of gravity is greatly reduced by the buoyancy force of water, the pregnant women will often find that her body alignment (posture) improves while submerged in the water. The weight of the developing fetus tends to create excessive lordosis, and the increase in breast size tends to round the shoulders forward - the buoyant environment allows the woman to return to a more neutral position comfortably. Exercising in the water is safe and effective and will improve, or at the very least maintain, muscular strength and endurance as well as cardio-respiratory endurance. Exercise during pregnancy - just as any other time in a woman's life - helps to maintain energy levels, reduces stress and fatigue, and creates an overall positive attitude.

Certain precautions must be taken by pregnant and post-partum women during exercise to protect their health and the health of the unborn fetus. Some of these precautions were briefly discussed previously; it is advised to become more adequately trained in this area before developing a perinatal program of your own.

CROSS TRAINING

Variety may very well be the key to exercise adherence. Variations in workouts not only prevent boredom and burnout, but allow for greater gains, aids in overcoming training plateaus, and can help prevent injuries - both from overtraining and from muscular imbalances. Cross training - developing physical fitness by training in more than one activity - is gaining acceptance by the professional athlete as well as the general population.

The book, *Cross Training: Ultimate Fitness* by Time-Life Books, compares three sports conditioning activities and the muscles that each one utilizes to show the benefits of cross training in developing a total-body regimen. These three sports - swimming, cycling, and running - compliment each other in the type of workout provided. These comparisons are summarized in the chart on page 63.

Aquatic exercise programs offer an ideal method of cross training for many people. Runners are learning that by alternating their traditional training program on land with deep water running, they can actually improve their competitive times. Bodybuilders utilize aquatic aerobic exercise to improve muscular definition before competition. Sports-specific aqua programs provide seasonal cross training workouts that can be designed to benefit individual team members or the group as a whole. The general population benefits by having an option to land aerobic classes that offers comparable benefits to aerobic training with increased resistance to muscular system and less stress to the joints.

ACTIVITY	PRIMARY MUSCLE GROUPS	SECONDARY MUSCLE GROUPS
Swimming	Latissimus dorsi Triceps Deltoids Pectoralis major	Quadriceps Abdominals
Cycling	Gluteus maximus Quadriceps	External obliques Latissimus dorsi Erector spinae Trapezius Wrist extensors
Running	Soleus Gastrocnemius Hamstrings Quadriceps	Gluteus maximus Abdominals Trapezius

REHABILITATION

Water has long been known for its therapeutic benefits; hydrotherapy can range from a muscle-relaxing soak in a whirlpool to an extensive, supervised physical therapy program to meet specific goals. The water environment often allows individuals to move without the pain experienced on land, because they are no longer working against gravity. Most participants will find it is easier to move the joints through a greater range of motion while that particular body part is submerged in the water.

Pool temperature for therapeutic programs is generally recommended to be above the 80-84 degree range suggested for general population exercise classes. According to Barry Deuel, A.T.C., at the Medical Circle Physical Therapy and Sports Medicine Clinic, the temperature depends upon the individual patient's needs. He suggests that when working with geriatric patients in a rehabilitative or conditioning program (not aerobic in nature) the water be approximately 88-92 degrees Fahrenheit; being cooler than body temperature, this will stimulate participants to move and yet still be comfortable for low-intensity exercises. Working with younger patients under a similar program, the water can be tolerated at lower temperatures (80-85 degrees). Another consideration is the facility itself; many pools are multi-functional, and a mid-range for all clients must be maintained.

The Arthritis Foundation is an excellent source of information for more advance training when developing an aquatic program geared toward arthritic clients. It is recommended that the pool temperature be approximately 86 degrees Fahrenheit when conducting a class for participants with arthritis. Cooler water temperatures can aggravate the joint inflammation and cause discomfort during and after exercise. The main focus of this type class is to develop and maintain normal range of motion at the joints. Other special populations and suggestions for water temperatures for exercise are as follows: multiple sclerosis (80-84), muscular dystrophy (90-95), cerebral palsy (cool water temperatures may limit movements), asthma (indoor pools are usually preferred to avoid extreme temperature changes). It is generally suggested that air temperature be within 5 degrees of water temperature when working with special populations.

MUSIC

Music is optional for conducting an aquatic exercise class, although many instructors and participants feel that it is a critical component for motivation. Poor acoustics and background noise (fans and pump systems as well as other participants in the area) often associated with pool facilities may prevent the use of music; if the music becomes a hindrance rather than a help it should be eliminated. Some facilities do not allow music to be used at the pool area for various reasons, and management policy must be followed. Whichever method of teaching you choose, or are assigned to, can be effective, but some considerations for selecting music are discussed below.

BEATS PER MINUTE

Most aquatic exercise instructors prefer music of approximately 130-150 beats per minute (bpm) for the aerobic warmup and training segment of class in general populations. This is a similar tempo to what is commonly utilized in low impact land aerobic classes. It is important to remember that when using music of this speed in an aquatic class, that you count every other beat per minute to compensate for the decreased speed of movement in the water. Music of 120 bpm or less can sometimes be used at tempo, depending upon the movements. Toning exercises work well with music approximately 110 bpm.

Instructors working exclusively with older adults often recommend a slower tempo due to the decreased reaction time of the participants. Music of 115-130 bpm usually is suitable.

Tapes designed for bench aerobic classes usually fall within the 118-126 bpm range and so are ideal for various water aerobic programs. To perform aquatic bench stepping classes, however, the tempo should probably be lowered to about 110 bpm for most individuals and allow for correct foot placement and body alignment.

Do not completely limit yourself to music that is within a specified tempo; if you like a song, experiment with it and likely you can find a use for it in your exercise program. Although pre-mixed aerobic tapes are usually designed to provide a steady increase, peak, then decrease in bpm, it is okay if you choose to intermix music of different speeds as long as the overall goals of your class are not compromised.

TYPES OF MUSIC

Music selection should first be based upon the preferences of the class participants, and secondly that of the instructor, to be most effective. An instructor must enjoy the music style in order to be creative and enthusiastic, but if the students are not satisfied, they may not return. Most class participants are more than willing to provide feedback on music preferences if given the opportunity.

Besides the pre-mixed low-impact aerobic tapes available, try music styles such as Christian, country, big band era, Broadway, classical, jazz, and top forty. Theme tapes for special occasions such as Halloween, Christmas, and the Fourth of July can also be a fun way of incorporating non-traditional music in your aqua fitness class. Instrumental may be more appropriate to classes with older adults; the lyrics can often make it more difficult for the participants to hear the instructor's verbal commands. Music can definitely enhance an exercise class, especially if the choreography is appropriate.

MUSIC RIGHTS

The 1976 U.S. Copyright Law states that music may be a copyrighted entity, and if so, requires the user to obtain permission for use and to pay royalties for any public performance. Virtually all facilities where music is played, even as "background" music, are subject to the law. The American Society of Composers, Authors and

Publishers (ASCAP) and BMI are the two largest music licensing organizations. Both organizations will provide a music performance agreement for yearly fee based on the size of the business; this agreement entitles the member business to play any of the specified music an unlimited number of times throughout the year.

The facility is responsible for paying the royalty fees as the yearly charge is based upon the number of participants or the square footage of the facility. All instructors who teach at the location would be covered. However, if an instructor is an independent contractor, he or she may be responsible for paying this fee. Music that is considered to be public domain is not covered by the Copyright Law and can legally be used without paying the user fees. However, be aware that some newer arrangements of this music may be copyrighted.

SUGGESTED SOURCES

Some suggested sources for music to utilize in your aerobics classes are as follows:

STROM-BERG PRODUCTIONS (original music)
1-800-82-TUNES

DAVID SHELTON PRODUCTIONS (offers many theme tapes)
1-800-272-3411

AEROBIRHYTHMS (Christian music) = 817-294-1222

IN-LYTES PRODUCTIONS = 1-800-243-PUMP

FIT NET = 1-800-288-BFIT

MUSCLE MIXES = 1-800-52-MIXES

DYNAMIX MUSIC SERVICE
203 Edgevale Road
Baltimore, MD 21210

POWER PRODUCTIONS = 1-800-777-BEAT

TWELVE INCH DANCE RECORDS = 1-202-659-2011

THE ENERGY DIVISION = 1-800-488-4NRG

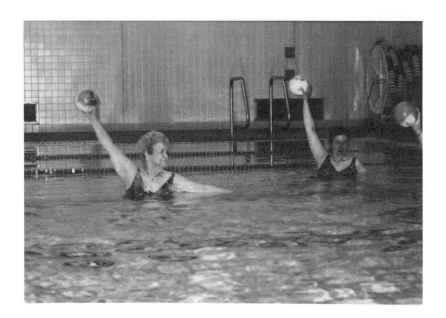

ARM POSITIONING

One of the most debated topics in aquatic exercise is whether to utilize the arms under or above the water surface. The authors feel strongly that the majority of the arm movements should be performed under the surface of the water during the aerobic and toning portions of class. We have moved aerobic classes into the pool environment because of the beneficial properties of water; it seems contradictory, therefore, not to take advantage of these special qualities. If the arms are held above the water's surface, we cannot receive the toning benefit provided by the water's extra resistance.

Many instructors and participants believe that they cannot obtain an intense workout with the arms submerged. Usually this thinking is due to the fact that the person is not adequately acquainted with water exercise principles. The intensity depends upon many factors, including how much force the individual exerts with each movement, the length of the lever arm, the frontal surface area, and eddy drag. All of these factors can easily be manipulated with changes in arm and hand positioning, thereby increasing or decreasing the intensity of the workout. The water feels so good, that sometimes it is possible to "go with the flow" rather than work against the water; in swimming skills we want to be very efficient in our movement through water, but in aquatic exercise we must make the movements less streamlined and more inefficient, so to speak, to gain the maximum intensity levels.

Another misconception is that the heart rate is strictly tied to the aerobic intensity. Remember from previous discussions of heart rates (Chapter III) that this in not completely true; we use the heart rate as a means of monitoring intensity because it is easy and a fairly accurate guideline in most individuals. But heart rate will be affected by many other factors besides the intensity of the aerobic workout. While the heart rate will surely be elevated if the arms are utilized overhead for an extended period of time, this does not represent a similar metabolic response. An analogy which may prove helpful is: if you measure your pulse while watching a scary movie, you will find that it is elevated above your resting heart rate and possibly into your target zone - this does not however qualify for aerobic exercise.

Finally, arm movements maintained in a flexed position for a sustained period of time will cause unnecessary stress to the shoulder joint. Exercise programs should be designed to improve fitness levels, not hinder improvements or create injury. Some arm movements out of the water, and above the head, are needed to provide movement through the body's full range of motion. Some arm movements out of the water are beneficial for variety and creating certain styles of choreography. Some arm movements out of the water should be included. Avoid teaching, or participating, in an aquatic exercise program where the arms remain exclusively above the water's surface.

SAMPLE PROGRAMS

Basic, sample programs will be given for beginner, intermediate, and advanced level aqua aerobic exercise, as well as a modification for working with an older adult population. This is not designed to teach specific exercise routines, but rather to explain general sequencing for an effective program. Individual modifications, and preferred steps and combinations, are to be added by the instructor to develop a personalized program. These programs assume that the participants represent an average, general population with no medical problems that would inhibit their participation; water temperature and depth are as previously recommended for shallow water aerobic exercise.

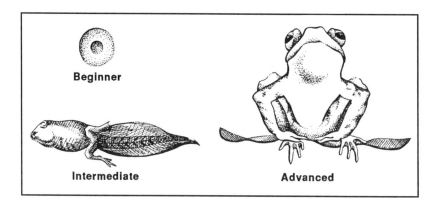

Beginner

Intermediate

Advanced

BEGINNER LEVEL
(TOTAL CLASS TIME 45 - 50 MINUTES)

Thermal Warm-Up (3 - 5 minutes)

Water walking while traveling in circles, across pool, following lane lines etc; vary the arm and leg movements so that all the major muscle groups are utilized; travel forward, backward, and laterally or if space is limited the following should be considered:

- Stationary gentle bouncing or bobbing with feet together, apart, and alternating; arms may push towards bottom, front, sides, or overhead.
- Easy jog or march in place with knees high and heels high; arms swinging front to back at the sides keeping the elbow slightly flexed and fingers slicing through the water.

Pre-Stretch (3 - 5 minutes)

Static stretches, in combination with rhythmic stretches if desired, for the following muscle groups: calf, tibialis anterior, hamstrings, quadriceps, hip flexor, buttocks, lower back, upper back, chest, shoulders, and neck; hold the stretches.

Cardio Respiratory Warm-Up (3 - 5 minutes)

Easy jog or march with heels high and travel forward incorporating front crawl arm movements; reverse, and travel backwards with knees high and back crawl arms.

Slow water speed movements such as knee lifts, cross country skiing, and jumping jacks; 16-32 repetitions of each before changing exercise.

Cardio Respiratory Training (20 minutes)

Increase the intensity of the movements by incorporating fast water speed steps, utilizing long levers (kicks instead of knee lifts for example), and performing only 8-16 repetitions before changing exercises.

Incorporate traveling patterns if space permits; include lateral travel, such as crossing steps and side steps, as well as forward/ backward movements.

Vary the hand positioning and lead with the palm to increase the intensity - a slightly cupped palm will provide the greatest resistance.

Exercise continuously for the 20-minute period at about 50-65% of the heart rate reserve, or at a "somewhat hard" level of perceived exertion.

Toning and Strengthening (10 minutes)

Choose from the following:

Standing at a depth where the shoulders can be submerged if possible, perform exercises for upper body muscle groups; work in a slow and controlled manner - remember that pulling the water with a slightly cupped hand will provide the greatest amount of resistance; not all upper body muscles need to be exercised specifically in each work-out, but be sure to exercise opposing groups during the same workout (biceps and triceps for example).

Moving to the pool edge for support and perform exercises for lower body muscle groups; work in a slow and controlled manner; keep the supporting leg slightly flexed to prevent stress to the knee and avoid hyperextending the lower back; not all lower body muscles need to be exercised specifically in each workout, but be sure to exercise opposing groups during the same workout (hamstrings and quadriceps for example).

Utilizing flotation equipment (hand-held, around the upper arms or around the torso); perform abdominal exercises from a supine position; remember that abdominal "crunches" work most effectively if the movement is initiated with the shoulders (pulling the knees to the chest primarily utilizes the hip flexors) and that adding a twist will incorporate the obliques; also remember to breathe normally and do NOT hold the breath.

Final Stretch (5 - 10 minutes)

Perform static stretches for the major muscle groups, especially those muscles specifically exercised during the toning/strengthening segment; hold the stretches about 15-30 seconds.

Be sure to spend ample time stretching the gastrocnemius and soleus (calf muscles).

INTERMEDIATE LEVEL
(TOTAL CLASS TIME 60 MINUTES)

Thermal Warm-Up (3 - 5 minutes)

Water walking and/or jogging while traveling in circles, across pool, following lane lines etc; vary the arms and leg movements so that all the major muscle groups are utilized; travel forward, backward, and laterally or if space is limited the following is an alternative:

- Stationary bouncing or bobbing with feet together, apart, and alternating; arms may push towards bottom, front, sides or overhead.
- Easy jog in place with knees high and heels high; arms crossing front and back keeping the elbow slightly flexed and hands relaxed.
- Cross country skiing in place; arms swinging front to back at the sides keeping elbows slightly flexed and hands relaxed.

Pre-Stretch (3 - 5 minutes)

Static stretches, in combination with rhythmic stretches if desired, for the following muscle groups: calf, tibialis anterior, hamstrings, quadriceps, hip flexor, buttocks, lower back, upper back, chest, shoulders, and neck; hold the stretches.

Cardio Respiratory Warm-Up (3 - 5 minutes)

Jog with heels high and travel forward incorporating breast stroke arm movements; reverse, and travel backwards with knees high and reversed breast stroke arms.

Intermix slow and fast water speed movements such as knee lifts, kicks, cross country skiing, and jumping jacks incorporating specific arm movements.

Cardio Respiratory Training (30 - 35 minutes)

Increase the intensity of the movements by exerting more force - work against the water's resistance and elevate the movements by bouncing higher.

Incorporate traveling patterns if space permits; include lateral travel, such as jumping jacks and sliding, as well as forward/backward movements, such as leaping.

Include some higher impact moves such as tuck jumps, frog jumps, and straight jumps; elevate as high out of the water as participants are able to perform.

Lead with the palm to increase the intensity - a slightly cupped palm will provide the greatest resistance; webbed gloves will provide further resistance.

Exercise continuously for the 30 minute period at about 65-75% of the heart rate reserve, or at a "somewhat hard" to "hard" level of perceived exertion.

Toning and Strengthening (10 - 15 minutes)

Choose from the following:

Standing at a depth where the shoulders can be submerged if possible, perform exercises for upper body muscle groups; work in a controlled manner increasing the speed as strength gains are made; addition of resistance equipment will provide additional gains; not all upper body muscles need to be exercised specifically in each workout, but be sure to exercise opposing groups during the same workout (biceps and triceps for example).

Performing "power moves" for lower body muscle groups; work in a slow and controlled manner to isolate various muscle groups; addition of resistance equipment will provide additional strength gains; not all lower body muscles need to be exercised specifically in each workout, but be sure to exercise opposing groups during the same workout (hamstrings and quadriceps for example).

Utilizing flotation equipment (hand-held, around the upper arms or around the torso); perform abdominal exercises from supine and vertical (if water depth is sufficient) positions; hand- held flotation equipment can also provide additional resistance by pulling under the knees during the "crunches."

Final Stretch (5 - 10 minutes)

Perform static stretches for the major muscle groups, especially those muscles specifically exercised during the toning/strengthening segment; hold the stretches about 15-30 seconds.

Be sure to spend ample time stretching the gastrocnemius and soleus (calf muscles).

ADVANCED LEVEL
(TOTAL CLASS TIME 60 - 75 MINUTES)

Thermal Warm-Up (3 - 5 minutes)

Jogging and power striding while traveling in circles, across pool, following lane lines etc; vary the arm and leg movements so that all the major muscle groups are utilized; travel forward, backward, and laterally or if space is limited do the following:

- Stationary bouncing or bobbing with feet together, apart, and alternating; arms may push towards bottom, front, sides or overhead.
- Jog in place with knees high and heels high; arms crossing front and back, keeping the elbow slightly flexed and hands relaxed.
- Cross country skiing in place; arms swinging front to back at the sides keeping elbows slightly flexed and hands relaxed.

Pre-Stretch (3 - 5 minutes)

Static stretches, in combination with rhythmic stretches if desired, for the following muscle groups: calf, tibialis anterior, hamstrings, quadriceps, hip flexor, buttocks, lower back, upper back, chest, shoulders, and neck; hold the stretches.

Cardio Respiratory Warm-Up (3 - 5 minutes)

Jog with heels high and travel forward incorporating breast stroke arm movements; reverse, and travel backwards with knees high and reversed breast stroke arms.

Intermix slow and fast water speed movements such as knee lifts, kicks, cross country skiing, and jumping jacks incorporating specific arm movements.

Cardio Respiratory Training (45 - 55 minutes)

Increase the intensity of the movements by exerting more force - work against the water's resistance and elevate the movements by bouncing higher.

Incorporate traveling patterns if space permits; include lateral travel, such as jumping jacks and sliding, as well as forward/backward movements, such as leaping.

Include an interval training segment of 10-20 minutes, alternating between higher impact moves (such as tuck jumps, frog jumps, straight jumps, straddle jumps on the wall, "climbing the wall," and "power jacks") to elevate heart rates to upper limit, and lower impact "power" moves to provide adequate lower body strengthening and toning during the aerobic segment.

Utilize webbed gloves to provide upper body strengthening and toning during the aerobic portion of class; make the arm movements precise and controlled.

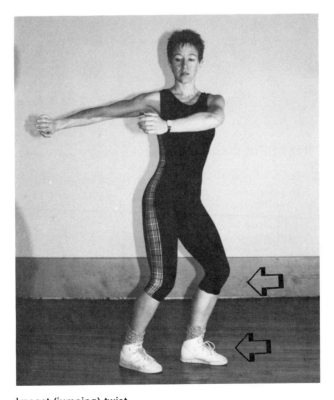

Impact (jumping) twist

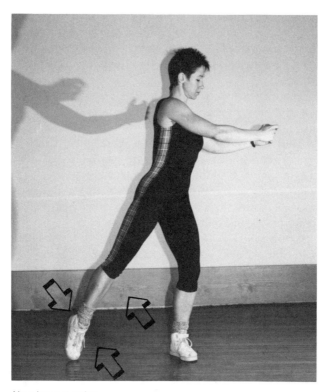

Non Impact twist

Toning and Strengthening (5 - 10 minutes)

Utilizing flotation equipment (hand-held, around the upper arms or around the torso), perform abdominal exercises from supine and vertical (if water depth is sufficient) positions; use hand-held flotation equipment to provide additional resistance by pulling under the knees during the "crunches."

Final Stretch (5 - 10 minutes)

Perform static stretches for the major muscle groups, especially those muscles specifically exercised during the toning/strengthening segment; hold the stretches about 15-30 seconds.

Be sure to spend ample time stretching the gastrocnemius and soleus (calf muscles).

REFERENCES

Cross Training, Ultimate Fitness. Alexandria, VA: Time-Life Books, 1988.

Horstmeyer, Barbara. *Perinatal Certification Instructors Manual.* Milwaukee: Maternity Fitness, Inc.

Deuel, Barry, A.T.C. Medical Circle Physical Therapy and Sports Medicine Clinic, Winchester, VA. July, 1991.

The Aquatic Exercise Association Instructor Certification Program, Aquatic Exercise Association, Port Washington, WI.

Chapter 4

THE OLDER/
MATURE ADULT

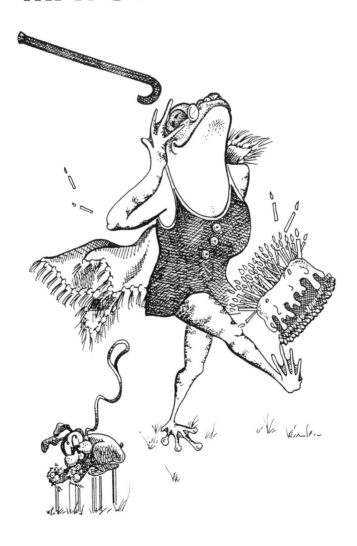

EFFECTS ON AGING

If a person has not participated in a regular exercise program for an extended period of time, and especially if he or she has led a sedentary life, his or her fitness level in most cases, will be on the low side of the scale. Older adult individuals do not necessarily fall into a special population of exercise participants, and there is no pre- determined age where we must adjust our fitness program to a different level. As the human body ages, certain changes do occur that may impact our life-styles, as well as our exercise program.

Ciscar and Kravitz writing in "Idea Today" discussed five primary biological effects of aging.

1. Although weight may stay the same or decrease somewhat, the percentage of body fat increases. A higher proportion of fat tends to be stored in the abdominal area, and this can be related to various metabolic disorders.
2. Muscle mass decreases due to atrophy of the fibers and a decrease in number of fibers.
3. Bone mass decreases and is closely linked with osteoporosis. A change in connective tissue (tendons and ligaments) leads to a decreased range of motion.
4. Aerobic and anaerobic capacities are reduced
5. Psychomotor control tends to decline leading to slower reaction times and difficulty with balance.

It has been documented that regular exercise, including aquatic programs, can play an important part in "slowing down" the aging process in numerous ways. Aerobic exercise can help to prevent heart disease by strengthening the heart, the lungs, and the circulatory system, by improving body composition and by altering the cholesterol levels to a more suitable ratio. Exercise not only keeps the body mobile through improvements in muscular strength, muscular endurance, and flexibility, but it helps also to strengthen the bones which normally become less dense with age. Other benefits include regulation of blood sugar levels and control of blood pressure.

The body, and all of its systems, are susceptible to the process of reversibility ("if we don't use it, we lose it" syndrome). Older adults who have led sedentary lives for several years will see an overall decrease in fitness level and, in turn, a greater difficulty in performing daily tasks. Often, if this pattern is not altered, the person will find himself or herself completely dependent upon others; since this reversibility process occurs in all systems of the body, mental, emotional, and physical abilities can be impaired. The pool can become a suitable location for exercise programs which encourage independent, productive, and happy lifestyles among the elderly.

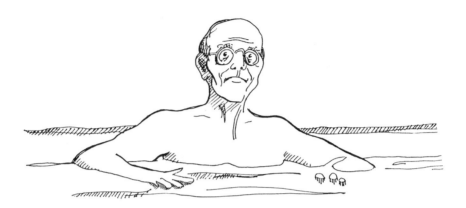

BENEFITS OF EXERCISE

"I was injured in an auto accident and suffered a broken pelvis and hip joint requiring a hip replacement. I took months of physical therapy and daily routine of exercise prescribed by my doctor. He also recommended a water exercise program, but due to the required 80 mile trip, I was unable to participate in the program."

"I joined Julie See's water aerobics program and in less than four weeks I made a marked improvement. This water aerobic routine not only strengthened my muscles in the leg and hip which had been injured, but improved my muscle tone and coordination, helping me overcome my limp. This improvement was acheived without muscle soreness or stiffness. I recommend the water aerobic program very highly."

Christine Maxwell

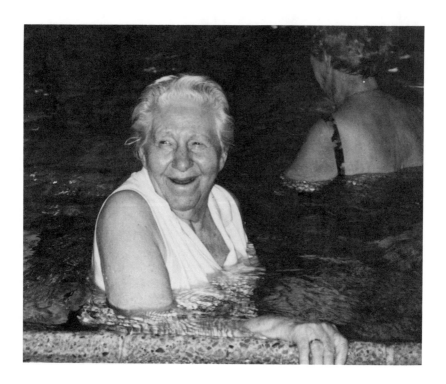

The older adult is a fast-growing segment of the American population, and it is a segment that all of us are approaching - because aging is not selective. Therefore, by becoming involved in a regular exercise program at a young age, by encouraging others to develop this same lifestyle, and by developing and providing older adult classes, we each have the ability to positively influence many individuals.

Many groups and individuals have chosen to specialize in the field of aquatic exercise for the older adult. Karl Knopf teaches an Older Adult Aquatic Certification program which focuses on the physiological changes that occur with aging, and how to develop aquatic exercise programs to compensate for these changes. Sandy Stoub, a fitness specialist and the director of Essert Associates, Inc., has spent a great deal of time and energy in designing and implementing classes that focus on the specific needs of the older adult exercise participant, both land and water programs. Stoub recommends the major goal of an older adult class is to promote "functional fitness," or the ability to perform daily tasks with ease and comfort. As with any special population group, there are certain precautions to be taken. With older adults, Stoub suggests including an active warm-up period immediately upon entering the water to prevent participants from becoming chilled, altering the muscle groups being exercised more frequently to prevent fatigue, and being cautious with directional changes which can be confusing and difficult. Classes also should encourage postural improvements through well-designed choreography. As with any group, the class atmosphere set by the instructor is very important; with older adults do not forget the element of fun, include lots of praise, and remember to speak with respect (most people do not like to be referred to as "honey" and "deary" - except maybe from their spouse).

A medical clearance to participate in class is advised, and a medical history on each participant should be in a convenient location for quick reference. Of importance to note is the use of medication(s) and past surgeries. For example, participants having had hip replacement surgery should avoid crossing the midline of the body with the leg, and added resistance should be used with extreme caution for women having had a mastectomy. If a participant requires medication, especially for an illness which can be impacted by exercise, such as heart disease or asthma, it may be advisable for that person to bring the prescription to class with them in case of an emergency.

Basically the GENERAL CLASS FORMAT discussed previously can be followed when designing programs for older adult participants. However, a longer warm-up should be included to properly prepare the joints for more strenuous use. General recommendation would be to limit the aerobic segment to 20-30 minutes at a low-impact level to avoid excessive stress and fatigue. Monitoring heart rates is often best accomplished through perceived exertion due to the difficulty in counting pulse rate and the prevalence of medication use by participants. Specific muscular strengthening exercises to improve body alignment are important to include, possibly in the toning segment as well as in the choreography of the aerobic segment. In addition, special attention should be given to stretching to promote long-term flexibility. Not only will this facilitate performance of daily activities, but it also will allow for improvements to postural deviations associated with aging.

For example, kyphosis is an increase in the thoracic curve of the spine and is often noticed in older adults, creating a "hunchback" appearance. This may be due to degeneration of the spinal column as well as muscular imbalance. A properly designed exercise program can increase bone density and improve joint stability in the spine, strengthen the muscles in the upper back (trapezius, rhomboids, and posterior deltoids), and stretch the muscles in the front of the upper body (anterior deltoids and pectoralis). For an individual with pronounced kyphosis, this type of exercise program may provide for an improvement in the degree of curvature of the spine, and it may prevent, or slow down, the

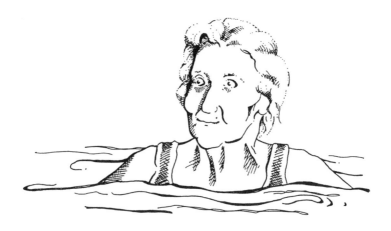

occurrence of this postural deviation in other individuals. An added benefit of exercise in the water is that the gravitational pull on the body is decreased, allowing the body to assume better postural alignment which may not be possible on land.

An added benefit of any exercise program is mental and emotional well-being. Exercise can reduce stress and tension, improve self-image, provide social interaction, decrease insomnia, and stimulate the mental capacity of participants. For the older adult, an exercise class can be a much-needed opportunity for human companionship. An individual who has lost his or her spouse, lives alone, and has no family members living close by may spend an entire day without talking to, much less touching, someone; for those persons, choreography that incorporates "touching" movments may be a welcome change. Some of the minor components of physical fitness - balance, agility, and coordination - should be directly addressed in an exercise program as well. These are psychomotor skills and therefore normally exhibit a decreased response as an individual ages. Choreography that gradually increases movements which require the use of mental as well as physical resources will be beneficial to the participants. For example, including steps which require the arms to move in opposition to the legs, reversing direction of travel, and challenging participants to recall the sequence of exercises with add-on choreography will help to develop coordination skills. You can encourage improved response times with pyramid choreography which first teaches a series of steps with many repetitions and then sequentially decreases the numbers of repetitions of each step. Balance may be enhanced by incorporating standing leg exercises and stretches in the center of the pool instead of along the side of the pool. Plan your program to give the most possible within the time limits of each class and freely give praise and encouragement to each participant.

PROGRAMMING FOR AQUATICS

Given below a sample class format for programs designed for an older adult population; as with any class, individual modifications will be necessary and the pool conditions (water depth, water and air temperature, slope of pool bottom, etc) must be considered. Music, if used, should be appropriate for the participants - in tempo, style, and volume.

TOTAL CLASS TIME (45 - 50 MINUTES)

Thermal Warm-Up (5-10 minutes)

Water walking while traveling in circles, across pool, following lane lines etc; vary the arm and leg movements so that all the major muscle groups are utilized - begin with short levers and small range of motion, then increase length of levers, and finally increase to full range of motion; travel forward, backward, and laterally.

Note: the thermal warm-up may be an appropriate time for social interaction among participants; the instructor may use this time for finding out how each person is feeling that day and get to know new participants.

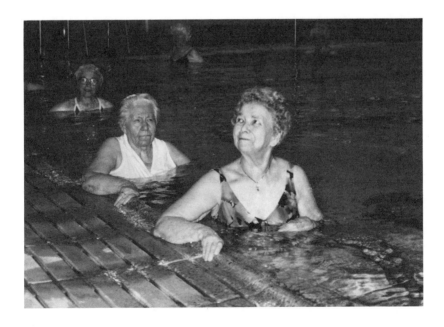

Pre-Stretch (3 - 5 minutes)

Static stretches, in combination with rhythmic stretches if desired, for the following muscle groups: calf, tibialis anterior, hamstrings, quadriceps, hip flexor, buttocks, lower back, upper back, chest, shoulders, and neck.

Prevent participants from cooling down during this segment of class by incorporating more vigorous movements between stretches, and by keeping the upper body moving during lower body stretches and vise versa.

Incorporate stretches and rythmic movements that take the arms overhead to maintain this range of motion through the shoulder joint.

Cardio Respiratory Warm-Up (3 - 5 minutes)

Easy jog or march with heels high, and travel forward incorporating front crawl arm movements; reverse, and travel backward with knees high and back crawl arms.

Slow water speed movements such as knee lifts, cross country skiing, and jumping jacks; 16-32 repetitions of each before changing exercise.

Cardio Respiratory Training (20 minutes)

Increase the intensity of the movements by incorporating fast water speed steps and utilizing long levers (kicks instead of knee lifts for example).

Incorporate traveling patterns if space permits; include lateral travel, such as crossing steps (caution those with hip replacement to modify) and side steps, as well as forward/backward movements; make sure that directional changes are well cued and slow enough for participants to safely follow; directional changes which require participants to have their backs to the instructor can be very confusing.

Vary the hand positioning and lead with the palm to increase the intensity - a slightly cupped palm will provide the greatest resistance.

Incorporate add-on and pyramid choreography techniques to develop agility and coordination; teach new steps and patterns slowly - teaching from deck is often very beneficial.

Exercise continuously for the 20-minute period at about 50-65% of the heart rate reserve, or at a "somewhat hard" level of perceived exertion.

Toning and Strengthening (5 - 10 minutes)

Choose from the following:

Standing at a depth where the shoulders can be submerged if possible, perform exercises for upper body muscle groups; work in a slow and controlled manner - remember that pulling the water with a slightly cupped hand will provide the greatest amount of resistance; not all upper body muscles need to be exercised specifically in each workout, but be sure to exercise opposing groups during the same workout (biceps and triceps for example); emphasize strengthening of the upper back muscles to improve posture.

Move to the pool edge for support and perform exercises for lower body muscle groups; work in a slow and controlled manner; keep the supporting leg slightly flexed to prevent stress to the knee and avoid hyperextending the lower back; not all lower body muscles need to be exercised specifically in each workout, but be sure to exercise opposing groups during the same workout (hamstrings and quadriceps for example); possibly incorporate some of these exercises without the pool edge for support to help develop balance.

Utilizing flotation equipment (hand-held, around the upper arms or around the torso), perform abdominal exercises from a supine position; remember that abdominal "crunches" work most effectively if the movement is initiated with the shoulders (pulling the knees to the chest primarily utilizes the hip flexors) and that adding a twist will incorporate the obliques; also remember to breathe normally and do NOT hold the breath.

Limit the number of repititions performed for each exercise and allow for rest periods as needed; stress the importance of proper body alignment.

Final Stretch (5 - 10 minutes)

Perform static stretches for the major muscle groups, especially those muscles specifically exercised during the toning/strengthening segment; hold the stretches about 15-30 seconds.

Be sure to spend ample time stretching the gastrocnemius and soleus (calf muscles), lower back, chest and shoulders.

Encourage relaxation and proper breathing techniques; avoid becoming chilled.

"COTTON EYE JOE"

Following is a choreographed routine that is suitable for older adult classes. It is a square dance adapted for the pool environment and is performed with partners so therefore incorporates some "touching" movements. Because of the speed of the music, it will be easier to first learn the routine without any music. Begin by teaching one pattern and repeating it many times until everyone is comfortable with the required movements before continuing on to the next pattern. Next practice all of the patterns in the sequence in which they are choreographed in the routine; except perform 8-16 repetitions of each one. Finally decrease the number of repetitions until you are performing the routine in sequence with the proper number of repetions for each pattern. (This is an example of pyramid choreography instruction.) After all of this is accomplished, add the music and increase the tempo.

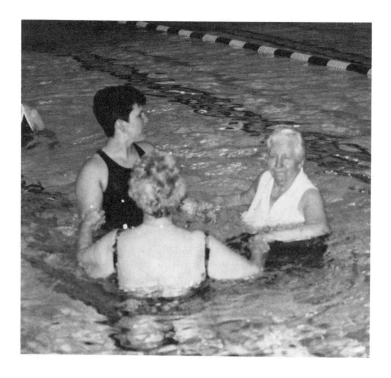

COTTON EYE JOE
Choreography by: Julie See

Wait 4 counts, lines facing partner

Pattern 1
Jog 4 in together/ jumping jack 2X
      (arms out, in, slap overhead, clap twice)
Repeat moving back
Jog in for 8, circle partner and jog back 8
      (arms crossed in front at chest height)
Repeat all of Pattern 1

Pattern 2
Promenade
      Jog in, join hands overhead; head of line moves between other
      couples to the tail of line while everyone else slides towards
      the head of line - end up where you began

Pattern 1
Repeat twice, first set of jog 4 stationary

Pattern 3
Swing your partner
      Jog in 8, hook right arms and circle 8; hook left arms and circle
      8, jog back 8 to opposite side from where you began

Pattern 1
Repeat twice

REFERENCES

Ciscar, Craig J. and Kravitz, Len. "Turning Back Time: Exercise and Aging." *IDEA Today* 9 (January 1991):28-35.

Stoub, Sandra. Director, Essert and Associates, Inc Consultants. Glen Ellyn,Illinois. August, 1991.

Chapter 5

EQUIPMENT

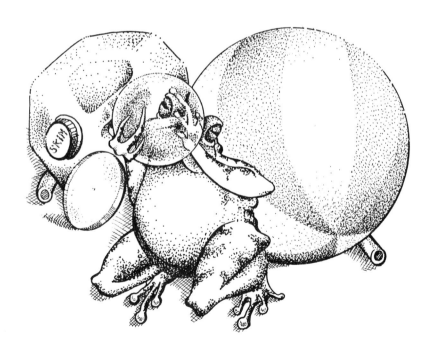

Although equipment is generally not necessary to conduct a safe, effective, and enjoyable aquatic exercise class, it can enhance an existing program or create an additional one. Equipment can provide additional resistance from the water (creating more frontal surface or eddy drag), increase buoyancy, or provide additional weight; therefore, greater gains in fitness levels can be realized by participants. Some groups of participants are more attracted to a class which utilizes equipment; you may increase the number of male participants in your aquatic program by incorporating special equipment. Equipment provides a source of variety for the participants and the instructor alike.

Deep water and aqua bench classes do require the use of special equipment. Deep water classes require flotation equipment so that participants can comfortably maintain proper body alignment while exercising; some flotation equipment also can provide added resistance during the workout. A specially-designed step is necessary to conduct aqua bench classes; keep in mind that not all bench-steps currently used in land aerobic programs will be suitable for use in the pool environment.

EQUIPMENT AVAILABLE ON THE MARKET

The variety, both in function and in cost, of aquatic exercise equipment available on the market today should suit most every need. Effective equipment can be purchased for under $10 per participant. In many cases, class participants are willing to purchase their own inexpensive equipment which further reduces the overhead cost of scheduling a class with equipment. Some of the general types of equipment currently used in aqua exercise classes include the following:

Flotation Belts - equipment designed to be worn around the waist for increased buoyancy; suitable for deep water programs and therapy

Flotation Vests - equipment designed to be worn on the torso for increased buoyancy; suitable for deep water programs and therapy

Ankle Cuffs or Boots - equipment designed to fit around the ankle to provide added flotation and/or resistance; variations in design including inflatable cuffs, buoyant foam cuffs, and neoprene boots with rigid plastic fins to provide resistance; suitable for deep and shallow water classes

Webbed Gloves - lightweight webbed gloves which are designed to increase the exercise intensity by providing a greater surface area of the hand which creates more resistance from the water; intensity variations are obtained by either slicing the hand through the water, making a fist, leading with the palm of the hand with fingers closed, or leading with the palm of the hand with fingers open; suitable for most any type of class and ability level

Dumbbells - dumbbells designed specifically for use in an aquatic environment which increase intensity through increased bouyancy, surface area, and/or eddy; some allow for variable resistance by making changes in the amount of surface area moved through the water; some are designed so that they may be filled with water instead of air - when used in this manner below the surface of the water, resistance is decreased, but when held above the surface of the water, resistance in increased; suitable for muscular strengthening and toning programs as well as appropriately designed aerobic activities

Paddles - rigid plastic paddles which increase the intensity of exercise primarily by increasing surface area of movement; may be attached to the palm of the hand or held in the hand; suitable for muscular strengthening and toning programs as well as appropriately designed aerobic activities

Exercise Bands - elastic bands which increase the resistance which the limb must move against - they do not rely on the properties of water for changes in intensity; can be utilized for upper and lower body exercises; most suitable for muscular strengthening and toning exercises

"HOMEMADE" EQUIPMENT

Many aqua instructors choose to utilize "homemade" equipment, usually because of limited funding. This type of equipment works along the same principles of buoyancy, surface area, and added weight to increase the intensity of a workout or to provide necessary flotation. One of the most common pieces of "homemade" equipment is the use of plastic jugs. When the cap is left intact, these jugs serve as flotation devices for vertical and supine movements, as well as added resistance for specific arm exercises when submerged. Another option is to cut the lower portion of the jug away, and holding by the handle, scoop the remaining part of the jug through the water for increased surface area. Some instructors partially fill the jugs with water; this will decrease the intensity of the workout when working with the jug submerged because the buoancy is lessened. Be very careful when using a partially filled jug above the water's surface because the weight is now unstable and could cause injury to the participant.

Plastic lids are sometimes incorporated into class for increased frontal resistance in specific arm exercises. By placing the lid in front of the palm, the force of the water will hold the lid in place while exercising as long as the participant leads with the palm during all directions of movement. No gripping is required, but exercises are limited.

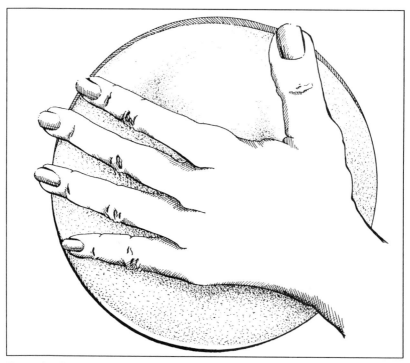

Example of "homemade" equipment - using plastic lid as a hand paddle.

SPECIAL CONSIDERATIONS

When incorporating any type of equipment into an exercise program, it is imperative that the instructor be fully trained and familiar with the equipment being used. The program must be designed around the specific equipment; not all equipment is suitable for all types of classes or all ability levels of participants. Equipment usually requires adjustment in speed and range of motion to ensure proper body alignment is maintained. New participants should be oriented to equipment function and proper techniques for utilization before beginning the first class.

When using plastic jugs as equipment, it is suggested that milk containers be avoided because of the possibility of contaminating the pool from bacteria which may be present if the jugs are not sufficiently cleaned. Also, remove all labels from the jugs before using in the pool, so that labels do not enter the filter systems.

If you select to incorporate equipment that is not specifically designed for aquatic exercise, for example milk jugs, you should take into consideration possible legal ramifications. Some authorities in the aquatic fitness industry believe that an instructor would more likely be found negligent in a court of law if the program included such "homemade" equipment than if the program were designed around equipment specifically developed for aquatic exercise.

Besides the legal considerations involved, an instructor may want to consider the degree of professionalism he or she hopes to convey through the class programming. Consider a health club that taught a strength training program that incorporated various sizes of stones instead of standardized free weights and equipment. One could develop a program, but would it be safe, effective, and professional? Would you, yourself, want to participate? It is not that "homemade" equipment is absolutely wrong, but it must fit the needs of your clients, your program, and your facility.

AQUA AEROBICS A Scientific Approach